The Fabric of Her Dancing Shoes

The Fabric of Her Dancing Shoes

by terri st. cloud

ISBN: 978-0-9815440-6-9
bone sigh books
www.BoneSighArts.com
www.BoneSighBooks.com

Cover art by Noah Urban
www.BFGproductions.com

contents

to the strands of
that testosterone filled gold
in my fabric -
bob.
josh.
noah.
zakk.
i love you guys.

i want my heart to open,
and open,
and open,
'cause i think god's in
there.

I can't figure life out. I'd like to. I think. Although, maybe I'd miss the pondering. For the past ten years of my life I've been knee-deep in a search. There have been moments I thought the search was to find myself, at other times it was to find the meaning of life or to figure out love. I've worked with many different slants and angles, but one theme seems to float continually throughout it all - the theme of 'real.' I want to find real. I want to find the real in me, I want to find the real in life, the real in love. I want real. Authentic, honest, non-delusional, real stuff.

Sometimes I feel like I can see things so clearly I can reach out and touch them. Other times I feel nothing but muddled and overwhelmed. Balance will come in once in awhile only to leave again shortly thereafter.

If you take a divorce and mix it up with an entirely new path in life, add several deaths that hit hard, some huge lessons in learning how to love, mid-life awakenings that shake the earth, empty nest beginnings that tug on the heart, beliefs shattering, beliefs growing, the blossoming of self worth, a tremendous amount of self doubt, body issues, mattering issues, a quick and vivid imagination, an appreciation of the feminine, a realization that there's something sacred swirling around, and some child-like wonder...you get a woman who has a lot of questions, very few answers, and a deep respect for the journey itself.

I have spent time with people who do have the answers. I don't like those times. It may be the answers that bother me, it may be the closed doors that those answers create that bother me. Whatever it is, I've come to enjoy being with people who are wondering and searching with me, who are okay with not knowing the answers and are open to thoughts all around them. It is in their company that I feel inspiration. It is in their company that I feel stronger and eager to explore what's happening inside of me. It is in their company that I become more.

There's inspiration in confusion. Perhaps it makes me feel less alone, perhaps it creates some sort of space for my thoughts to open and wander and discover. I'm not sure. I just know that I grow with questions more than I grow with answers.

There are no answers here. Just searching, pondering, confusion, delight, sorrow, and reaching. I've taken musings I have written earlier, added new thoughts as I went along, stitched them all together, gathered some loose ends, wove them into the mix and created this patch – a piece of my dancing shoes.

My dancing shoes are what I wear when I'm living fully, when I've joined in the dance of life. Those shoes are made from my heart's wonderings and my soul's longings. That is the fabric of my dancing shoes. And here, in these pages, are pieces of that fabric. I offer them to you. Maybe they can add a strand to your own weavings.

in and out,
up and down,
over and over,
she wove her strands of life together.
patching hole after hole.
eventually she saw it was more than
the threads that gave her strength,
it was in the very act of weaving itself
that she became strong.

*it's a powerful thing
to watch a woman wake up.*

Honor Yourself

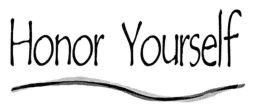

When I was 40, my life began to unravel. Sometimes I say it 'exploded.' It unraveled, exploded, fell apart, shattered, it changed. Drastically. I honestly believe this happened because I woke up to being a woman. I woke up to being a person. I woke up.

The waking up was like a birth. I feel like I gave birth to the woman I wanted to be. And then, once birthed, she needed to grow. Growing her...growing me...is going to be a life long process. The growing can take a lot of work at times. I find that I have to push myself to stretch myself. One of the biggest catalysts behind that pushing is my fear of falling back into the 'old ways.' Specifically denial. I wasn't just good at denial, I excelled at it. I was the Queen of Denial. I made denial a beautiful land full of happy things...only the happy things weren't real and they couldn't possibly feed my soul. You can't feed your soul with something not real. It scares me how easily and naturally I can play a game, how I can fall back into that kingdom. That fear of landing back there is one of the reasons I spend so much time looking at my thoughts and what I feel is really going on around me. I am on a quest to not only find real, I am on a quest to live real, and to stay real.

When I changed my world, I made a promise to the Universe. I would listen to my heart, I would follow what I heard, and I would live Love as best I could. That takes a whole lot of learning and UN-learning. There's a whole lot of overlap between topics. Life overlaps with power - inner power and power offered to the world, power overlaps with mattering - knowing you matter and living the fact that you matter, living the fact that you matter overlaps with inner child work, inner child work overlaps with self love, self love overlaps with rivers of steel and grace and trust and on and on it goes.

Logically sorting through all of this and laying it out in some coherent pattern seemed impossible. The fabric of my dancing shoes has no coherence. It's a delicious, sparkling, iridescent, deeply hued, woven, patched, glued, torn, tattered, strong, gorgeous fabric. It's a mish mash. Just like this book.

Mixing strands from my weaving, I hope to offer something that touches a place inside another that needs touching, that needs acknowledging and that needs honoring. I think that when we all start offering our strands, our weavings will get stronger and stronger and all of our dancing shoes will become lighter and lighter.

IT IS UP TO US
TO CREATE THE GOLD.
WE ARE OUR OWN
ALCHEMISTS.

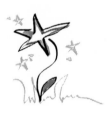

how to make
sense
out of the
ramblings...

When I was walking through some really dark hours, I discovered a tool that helped keep me sane. I wrote little snippets of what was whirling around inside me or around me. These snippets didn't really seem to fall into the category of poetry or quotes. Standing kind of in between those two worlds, they needed a name all of their own. Understanding that these weren't just part of me, but part of something bigger, part of some connection to something beyond me, I asked the Universe for a name. 'bone sigh' was what I heard. And that is what I call my poetry/quotes: 'bone sighs.'

Bone sighs have been weaving through my life for years now. They are the poetry-like quotes you see throughout the book. The different font is used to add a little funk to the mix and have them stand out on their own and to make you smile.

I had resisted the idea of writing a blog as I felt the world had enough noise in it already. It didn't need me to add to the din. And then one day, I got a note from someone that was filled with so much pain, I didn't know how to hold it all. That was the day I wrote my first blog. I put the pain and what I felt about it in the blog. I decided if I was going to keep it up and keep posting, then the only thing that I wouldn't consider noise would be ponderings of my own journey. Honest reflections of my quest to find real. And that is what I try to offer in my blog.

The sentences, paragraphs, and pages that are indented and set off with quotation marks are thoughts taken from that blog. They will refer to my daily walks and whatever was on my mind that day.

My thoughts written specifically for this book in an attempt to weave everything together with some sense of coherence are the sentences that go from margin to margin with no indentations.

You can read straight through just like any book or you can flip it open and start from wherever you are. There are no rules. Open your heart with me and come follow the meanderings.

i matter

it was when she first dared to
see her truth,
that the winds howled.
after a time,
it strengthened her
and she spoke her truth
and the earth shook,
and when finally,
she believed her truth –
the stars rejoiced, the universe
opened,
and even her bones sang her song:
"I Matter!"

The Beginning - I Matter!

'I matter' was the very first bone sigh I ever wrote. I'd like to say I wrote it when I figured out that I actually did matter. But to be quite honest, I had only figured out a tiny piece of that mattering. Someone once told me that I lived my way into my bone sighs. And I think that's true. I write them from glimpses I have inside of me, but it doesn't mean I have the concepts down and am living them yet. If I'm lucky, I grow my way into them.

Growing my way into mattering has been quite a long process. I lost a marriage, friends and family members on my journey into mattering. And while I see the beginning of that journey as the hardest time in my life, I cannot feel sad about it any more. What I gained from that time is more valuable to me than all that I lost. I gained myself. And you can't really have anything else until you have yourself, until you know that you are worthy and that you matter. The life I am building on that foundation is beyond anything I could have imagined. I absolutely rejoice in it.

My interactions with my self and with those around me have changed in deep ways, some subtle, some not so subtle.

"Why is it I forever want to make everything right for everyone?! Why?

I caught myself in that spot yesterday in such an outlandish way that it even made ME stop and shake me head! Then I found myself doing it again... getting ready to give something very important to myself away. It doesn't matter, I told myself. I can handle it and they'll feel better.

Woah. Hold up. Yeah! It DOES matter. And what does 'handling it' mean?? Getting through?? Is that what you want your life to be? Getting through? I thought you had enough of that?! Better look at this, Ter, because if you're ever going to really live a life of honesty and authenticity and believing you matter, you're choosing the wrong turn here.

So what is it? What's making you do these things?
I'm thinking it's the lack of trust, trust in several things...
Lack of trust in the other person to take care of themselves. Yeah, that's there. Lack of trust that it will end in a 'nice' way. Oh yeah, that's definitely there.

Lack of trust in myself...BINGO.

Am I really valuable enough to do what needs to be done to take care of me? Am I really valuable enough to say this isn't good for me, I'll just go over here where it's healthier? Am I really valuable enough to do the things that make me happy?

Hmmmmm...

But 'they' matter too. The other people. Shouldn't I take care of them too, the ones I'm trying to make it right for?

Maybe the best way of taking care of another person is living my truth, my real, my life, the healthiest way I can, and then allowing them the same, and leaving that up to them. Maybe that's respect for everyone.

That's all well and good until I have to interact with them. Then what do I say? What do I say when they say this or what do I say when they say that?

Hmmm...so is there fear that I can't be honest? Fear that I'll hurt them with my honesty? Fear that they'll say something to hurt me?

Yep.

Well, I can be honest. It probably will hurt them. And, yes, honestly, they will probably hurt me. So? What's the goal? To avoid hurt or to live real? To avoid hurt or to show all those little Terri's inside of you that they matter and you're going to stop setting them aside.

It's a deal. I know what I've got to do. As compassionately as I can, and as honestly as I can, with knowing that I matter, that all the parts of me matter...I'm going to take a walk in the rain and tell my 'little Terri's' that I choose them this time!

All I really have is me, I thought. I don't 'have' anyone else. It's me who needs to see this world of mine. It's me who needs to enjoy it. It's me who needs to live it."

Getting to the point where I could write that blog post took a lot of work. Some of the work I did was what I call 'Inner Child' work. Hence the references to the little Terri's. If it's a new concept, it can be an awfully strange one.

Someone recently told me that when her counselor spoke to her about working with her inner child, she didn't understand and the concept made her cringe. It's funny as when I first heard of the idea, I loved it. Wasn't sure what it was all about, but I plunged right on in there anyway. Anything that evokes a story or an image inside of me attracts my spirit.

I like to explain it this way. I have a friend who has something called Dissociative Identity Disorder or 'split personalities.' Having suffered repetitive trauma as a child, her way of protecting herself was to split into different personalities. I have learned so much from our conversations together about her experiences with her different parts. And through these conversations, I have come to believe that in a much, much, much milder form, we all have different parts inside of us. It can sound weird at first, but it really isn't strange at all. There's child like parts of us and adolescent parts of us, and frightened parts and all kinds of parts.

For me, actually visualizing them, putting faces and forms on them has become a tool that I've used to do some really powerful inner healing work. It's become one of my more delightful tools, and I talk about it enough now that my friends and family will actually refer to 'Little Terri.' I love that. It makes it all the more fun. You will see references to Little Terri throughout the book. Do not be alarmed. I have not lost my mind.

Visuals run rampant throughout the fabric of my dancing shoes. I love them. I'm not exactly sure why, but I can fall into them very easily and they turn out to be great tools to find out more about myself. I don't make them up as I go along. They just sort of take a life of their own inside of me. It's a bit like a dream, only I'm awake and they mostly make more sense more quickly to me than dreams do. While I love my dreams too and believe in working with them, I usually have to sit much longer with dreams to figure them out. These visuals I have while awake speak to me immediately.

"I had an awesome visual yesterday. I went way down to a deep level. To a place where not too many people have ever entered. And I found my shame. I didn't go there looking for it. I just kind of saw it there staring at me. Grumpy.

Odd, (or maybe not) it was in the form of a masculine snake. Nah, that's not so odd is it?

I was being guided through this visual. Someone was actually working with me as I told her what I was seeing. This was my first time for such a thing! She nudged me to ask what it was the snake wanted. I don't think I would have done that without being nudged. It had taken about all I had to figure out that he was my shame, but I thought it was a good question, and so I asked.

"To be loved," came the answer!

I laughed. You've got to be kidding me?! Does EVERYTHING want that?! Or maybe every PIECE of me does.

And so I did. I offered my love to the snake. And guess what? He morphed into a little girl then. A brilliantly beautiful little girl.

A thought occurred to me this morning. Loving my shame doesn't mean I love what happened to me. It means I love me. That might be worth re-typing.

Loving your shame doesn't mean you love what happened to you. It means you love you.

I don't know. That seemed like a new thought to me this morning. And it seemed like a real important little detail. Thought it was worth throwing out there..."

When I was about seven, I was molested. In the grand scheme of the horrible things that can happen to a person, I got lucky. It was only once. And it could have been a lot worse. BUT it affected me deeply. I think it has a lot to do with that shame that I went back and loved in my visualization.

> i went back and got her today.
> the little girl that is me.
> i coaxed her to stand,
> to drop the blanket,
> and to pick up her beauty.
> she's walking with me now,
> and leading me to wholeness..

"Almost every woman I know has had some kind of sexual abuse in her life. How astounding is that fact?! I am no exception. What part does that play in my life?

One day while working in my studio, without being anywhere close to thinking about when I was a child and was molested...it wasn't on my mind...I hadn't been thinking of it in the days prior...a thought landed in my head. Out of nowhere. It was this:

'That's when you figured out you didn't matter.'

Bam.
Just like that.
I even stopped what I was doing and looked up.
Huh?

But I heard it. And I knew what it meant.

That moment, so many years ago, affected me profoundly. I'm sure there's sexual repressions involved with that, but it's not just sexual. If it's when you feel you are told that you don't matter, how many different things get shoved down because of that? If you believe you don't matter, what do you hide away?

What if you believe you're different and don't fit in? Then what do you hide away? What parts of you do you cover so others won't see how different you really are?

Oh man.
As I thought about this, it almost got to be too much.
Wow!
I must have repressed most of me!

Here's the part that tickles me though, I want to go retrieve those parts. Yeah, I want to become more of who I am. As I typed that, a little tiny shot of fear ran through me. Yeah. The fear of rejection. You hide it away so as not to be rejected. You pull it out and what?

Yeah.
What?
I don't know. But I don't think I have a choice at this point. I think I've gone too far to turn back now..."

23

always with me,
waiting inside.
sometimes quietly,
sometimes not.
it is when i stop and listen
that i honor your presence.
it is when i follow what i hear
that i honor my wholeness.

It took me years and years to talk to anyone about what happened to me. And as I began, I heard more and more stories from women. The power of these moments is incredibly strong. I truly believe that going back inside ourselves, talking to our younger selves, holding those parts of us that need holding, and loving those parts is just as powerful a healing experience as those other moments were hurting experiences. Loving all of our selves is what leads us to wholeness.

tugging on my insides she asks me
to dance with her.
over and over she tugs.
finally, i notice.
finally, i turn to her.
holding no grudge for my being late,
she wraps her arms around my neck
and laughs in my ear.
it's time to dance, she says.
holding her in my arms,
we begin.

One of my favorite stories ever deals with a visualization that I spontaneously did with my inner child. I had gotten an email before I went out on my morning walk. It had a quote by Rumi in it that grabbed me by the veins. 'Forget safety. Live where you fear to live.' Oh my gosh, I thought that was so powerful. As I headed out on my walk, I decided I would find where it was I feared to live. I held different parts of my life to see if I was afraid of them. Nah, that one wouldn't feel right and I would try another. Somehow that's how I bumped into the idea that going back to the time when I was molested was something that really scared me. And that's how I decided to try a visualization.

So, as I walked, I went back in my mind. Now, truth be told, I have blocked a whole lot of it out of my memory. So going back accurately really wasn't possible. I had to wing it. Which is okay with me, I go more on feelings than details anyway.

I went back to the house it happened in. I pictured going down the hallway and walking up to a closed door. Opening the door, I found Little Terri sitting on the edge of a bed. She had a blanket wrapped tightly around her. Her head was bowed down. I could see my face looking at her. Every line, every detail of my face held such love for her. The tears poured down my cheeks. I went and sat next to her. Put my arm around her. Talked to her a little bit. Asked her if she'd come with me. She didn't want to. She didn't want to move. I coaxed her, coaxed her into dropping her blanket and holding my hand. We walked out of there together.

In a little while, I gave her a present. I had no idea what the present was. I just knew I had a brightly wrapped box for her. As she was opening it, I was peeking over her arm to see what was in there. She lifted out a framed picture of her and I sitting next to each other!

Later, walking towards home, I got ready to say goodbye to her. It hadn't occurred to me that she could stay with me. I was pretty new to these inner child visuals and just hadn't even thought of it. But then the idea hit me that she didn't have to go.

My gosh, she doesn't have to leave. 'Do you want to stay?' I asked her. And she did. We could stay together. Always. Hand in hand we walked into my house. And the feeling that she really was with me was so incredibly strong. I felt changed.

I thought about it later, and wondered if this story could help someone else. I decided to put it on our website. I felt totally shy and awkward about it, but the idea that it could help someone seemed to matter more. But if I was going to ask my sons to put it on our website, I should first tell my sons I was molested.

I have three sons. Sitting around our kitchen table, I looked at each of their faces. Ooooh this felt awkward. But I did it. I managed to get through the story. I didn't give a lot of details as no one needed those and then I told them about my walk and my visualization. I was so filled with it, that the story tumbled out, including the part about the gift.

My son, Noah, looked across the table at me and so gently told me that he could 'make that happen for me.' I didn't understand what he meant. He explained that he could combine a picture of me when I was little with one of me now. He could actually make the present become real. Tears rolled down my face again. What a gift. He did it, and it became a wallpaper for my computer. I use it whenever I need to remember that my inner child is right there next to me.

"I haven't a clue what any of this is about. All I know is that it feels like there's this whole treasure chest inside of me. But it's just too blurry yet to see...and that maybe my job is to see it."

"Who I am is all I have to offer. If it causes someone else discomfort, that's okay. That's not my deal. I can't take myself too seriously. And if opening is what I want to do, if that's what I want more than anything in the world, then I have to get up and keep going. And open. And so I'm here. And, yeah, I get points for being brave today. I'm putting the shame down. And I'm standing up and offering myself."

maybe offering something to the world is living
what you would want to offer.
maybe it's not any more than living it.
and maybe that's the hardest thing of all...

Offering is an idea that I really like. Everyone has gifts and strengths and something to offer the world. And if we all put those things out there, we could light the world on fire! Figuring out what exactly it was that I had to offer was driving me crazy though. I had my bone sighs and some people seemed really touched by them, but I still felt like I was missing something. I truly struggled with this one for a long time. Finally I came up with the idea that who I am was what I had to offer. I understood that my searching, my not knowing - my journey itself - was what I had to offer. I kept getting stuck on the idea that I needed to give answers and I had none. But as I thought about it, I realized that people's searching actually helped me a lot more than people's answers. Ha! I can offer confusion, I thought. I'm real good at that. And it felt right. Offer who I am. But in offering who I am, I have to know who I am, and I have to learn to really love who I am.

and the fist became the open hand.
she refused to beat herself any longer.
speaking words of kindness,
she gently touched her hair,
looked into her own eyes and
took the first step towards love.

"We're not crazy. We're not. We're not crazy. We're strong and resilient and growing and learning. It just doesn't feel that way so much sometimes. I don't know why it's so hard. It seems like it should be easy. I want something, why can't I just grab it with ease? But it's so hard sometimes.

But I chose now. I want to live now, to be now, to touch my authenticity now.

Every time I let the past close me down, every time I let the past dictate my actions, every time I let the past fill me with fear, I've lost that round.

Maybe it's not just that there comes a time when you have to decide what's going to win, the past or the present, maybe there comes a time when you have to commit to hanging in for all of the rounds and know that you are committed to winning more than losing. And maybe there comes a time when you have to decide you're worth the fight.

And maybe that brings you right back to the idea that there comes a time when you have to see your beauty, find your self love, and get up in the ring and know you can and will duke it out if you have to, because you are one unstoppable woman.

And maybe all that brings you to a time when deep in your cells you know you matter. Maybe your cells start carrying that message inside them, inside you.

And maybe those new cells outnumber the old cells.
And maybe there comes a time when you truly live.
Or maybe not.

Maybe there's never a 'time.' Only moments. Moment by moment you make the choice. Maybe it's millions and millions of opportunities to choose life. To choose yourself. To choose infinity. Over and over and over again.

Maybe that's actually a really cool deal. Maybe it's a gift you get a million trillion times in your life – the chance to choose you."

why do you look for it
over there?
the voice asked.
it's all inside you.
look within.
embrace what you see.
and dance with all that
is you.

All that is me...
I keep finding different parts to the 'all.' Sometimes I do believe it's endless...

Years ago an image came to me that captured my imagination. It was the image of a river running through me. With its color of steel and its strength of steel, it was obvious to me that this was my River of Steel. I had the idea that we all had one of these rivers inside of us. And when we found it, and touched it, we would remember our strength. I wrote this bone sigh from that image.

plunging her hands deep into
the mire,
she touched her river of steel.
shoving the muck
out of the way,
she let its silver waters
cleanse her.

It wasn't until later that I realized the river theme had been bubbling quietly inside of me for a long, long time. One of the first bone sighs I ever wrote, and one of my all time favorites, was based on the river image.

scratch the surface of her joy
and you will find a well of sorrow.
dive into the well and discover her spring of hope.
follow that spring to the river of her strength,
compassion and faith...
immerse yourself in her river and you will have
touched her soul.

Turns out rivers had been talking to me, and would continue to do so for years. The following thoughts filled my head as I walked one morning:

"There is a flow and we need to go with it. HOWEVER, a lot of that flow follows the grooves we carve. Being aware of those grooves is important. Constructing grooves that take things in a 'bad' direction is easy. It's the constructing of the 'good' grooves that takes a ton of work.

There is an inner river in all of us. Always. I'm just finding mine more and more. It's been there all along. Looking back, I can see it. It wasn't until I actually looked back and saw it that I started to feel it. Seeing it is key. Touching it often will remind me it's there and will feel like I'm growing it. But I think, actually, it will only open my eyes more and more to how big it has always been."

The water theme fit perfectly with the idea of the flow of life. I don't have any answers about how that works. What the 'flow' is, what that means, how you get in it or how you get out of it. But I do know that I've experienced it. I know there is something that you can step into where living becomes easier, where trusting becomes a way of life. I've had it. I've lost it. I've gotten it again. And lost it again. Over and over and over. But I have had it, I have touched it, I have danced in its waters. I know it exists.

"And as I walked, I thought of the love inside of me. I don't want it pushed out of me or stamped out of me, or anything out of me. I WANT that love inside of me. That ability to give love and believe in love and live love. But sometimes, I feel like it gets knocked right on out.

And then I remembered that river inside of me. I had been touching it daily. But the last few days, I hadn't touched it at all. It had been so easy to feel and reach before. I need to go find it, reach in and touch it and let it wash over me."

before it was like a drip she'd hear
now and then. not sure where it
came from or what it was about.
it wasn't until it became a stream
that she saw it. and now she knew it.
her river of strength, running thru her,
gaining power, growing fast and taking
her with it.

I think the image of water is powerful and can be used in so many ways to walk through what's going on inside of us. It can remind us that we have an inner core of strength. It can also help us remember that we can work with the things running through us. It is a part of us; we can touch it and we can direct it just as it directs us. There have been times when I feel overwhelmed with negative emotions, when I feel that everything running through me is going in the wrong direction, when my internal flow is heading down the wrong river bank.

"To try to stand up in a current that can feel overwhelming and to turn that current around, that's what I want to do.
I want to redirect the flow.
Yeah.
Redirecting the flow seems like it's going to take a lot of muscle.
But just imagine the raft ride afterward."

she sat with her toes in the water.
the little girl that is me.
sitting by my river of strength.
and i understood that they
were connected.
and i understood that my exploring
had only just begun.

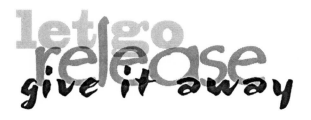

let go release
give it away

Control freaks come in many different forms and disguises. If you met me, you probably wouldn't consider me a control freak, but if you lived inside my head and watched the way I want to steer life and all the uncontrollable events, you might reconsider. That part of me that gets into a lot of the internal turmoil is my control freak side. I'm thinking I'm not the only one out there with this inside them. It's the part of me that gets angry when someone I love dies in a way that just doesn't seem 'fair.' Or the part of me that gets frustrated and wants to fix all my friends' problems, making their lives turn out beautifully. Or the part that worries about what's going to happen with a certain event, and doesn't want to let go into that flow of acceptance and knowing that whatever happens is okay. The part that screams 'NO! It's NOT okay!' That is my control freak side.

I spend a lot of time on my walks trying to get comfortable with the idea that I really have no control. The concept of trust is one of the biggest concepts I can embrace. To be honest, the true understanding of this lack of control has only really seeped in a handful of times. I know this because on those times, the realization knocked me to my knees. How terrifying it is to stare that truth in the eyes. Mostly, I say the words to show some comprehension of the idea, try to hold on to a fraction of what it means, and then work over and over and over again on learning this thing called trust.

Countless bone sighs have been written about trust, grooves have been worn in my street with all the walking and thinking I have done on this concept. And still, I wrestle with it constantly.

> "You can't hang on to this stuff. You can't control life. You can't make your life right, their life right, anyone's life right. You have got to let it go. But you've got to do more than let it go. You've got to give it away. You've got to give it away and trust. You've got to know it's all okay and give it away.
>
> And then when you do that, that's when you really feel alive. When you struggle, you're tense and stressed. When you stop struggling, then you're fatigued and worn out. The life energy isn't rolling through you. But when you sit and trust, and know it's okay, that's when you can finally feel alive. When you give it away, that's when you get it."

I'm not exactly sure what gets me to the point where I can finally give it away. Where I can finally let go. I know it happens, and I know I feel it when it happens, and it seems to come after a lot of struggle. But I really don't know what makes it so that I can release my grip. I do know that when I do release, the difference inside me is striking.

knowing she had to let go—
she released her grasp –
massaging her fingers
she reached for the possibilities
ahead of her.

maybe the holding stunts you,
she thought.
maybe growth is release,
non gripping, flowing,
ever forward, ever motion,
ever new...

radically accept release.
wildly desperately let go.
quietly hear the inner calm.
slowly, begin to know.

Letting go and releasing is tough for me in all areas of my life. Sometimes the business area is the place it's easiest for me to notice.

It's been a hard time for a small art business to stay afloat and keep things going, a time that has required a tremendous amount of trust, a time I haven't always had that trust. Sometimes the economics of the whole deal can really get me down. I think though that it's a choice I have to make. How am I going to handle the rough times?

"And then this morning, it hit me...business is slow. Get over it, Ter. That's okay. You can budget with the best of them. That's not your problem. You can handle that. But if you lose your intention, if you get wrapped up in the bummer part of it all, and forget what you're doing...well, then you're sunk.

If I lose my intention, I have nothing. It's real subtle and sneaks up on me and takes over me and I don't realize I'm losing it. But I see it now. And I want to hop in with both feet. Back to my intentions. Back into my belief in bone sighs. Back into knowing I'm going the right way, and just plowing through with delight.

Because that's what matters. If I don't have that, I might as well go get a real job. And so today, I turn back to my heart. And I let it free. And I follow it fully."

"If I know I'm doing what I've got to be doing, if I know I'm following my passion and listening to my heart, then sometimes I think I need to just pick myself up out of those pits of despair and go back to jumping in with both my feet. Getting out of the pit and back to the trust feels so good. There's magic in doing that, there's magic in how you walk, and there's magic in how you jump."

"I can't control who comes in and who leaves or when the bend changes or when the weather changes. Yeah, I hate that part. But it is what it is. All I can control is how I walk.

I felt kinda sad at one point today and I caught myself, reminded myself. It's HOW I walk. Sad's okay. It's not like I can't be sad. But throw in the trust. Walk in trust. Wrap all things in trust."

wrapping acceptance around her
entire being,
she stepped into trust.
entering the cathedral
of the truly living,
she watched the holy
take place.

more than anything –
i want to trust a journey
that i don't understand.

"As I walked up the next street, I thought of how hard I fight change. And how I want everything to be pretty.

It's not.

You wanted to be good and strong and happy today, Ter. Then step into that flow. Know that it's not all pretty and it changes constantly and deal with what's going on in the moments.

I want to enter my day open eyed to what's really there. Not what I want to be there. And truth is, today is filled with a lot of stuff that I don't want to be there.

But it is.
How I choose to live it is up to me. There are so many ways I run and hide. And I just don't want to do that anymore. I want to change 'run and hide' to 'step up and embrace.'

All of it. Every single bit of it.
And so once again, I turn to my day."

to lose myself in the dance so much so
that love will entangle my bones in its roots,
that when pain sears my heart,
courage will embrace the ashes
and wisdom will understand that it's all
part of the dance.

this is mine for the taking.
i pray my hands will grasp it,
my heart will open to it,
and i will know that i am the dance.

"I have to let my light shine, I thought. I really really have to. It's too foggy right now not to.

I walked, sang, and thought.

'That's it!' I thought. 'My gosh, that's it!'

I have been struggling for a week here trying to figure out how to be there for people right now. There's a lot of different people with a lot of different sadness. It seems everywhere I turn, the way they need me isn't my natural way. I struggle. And I try to bury my light.

Oh no. Oh no.

I can be there for them the way they need and still quietly shine my light. Still stay on the sidelines, holding up a candle, even if all that means is that I keep an awareness of light inside of me.

And then the visualizations started. I pictured some of the really hard times that I've been through with people. I went back to myself in each picture and I placed a candle in my hands. One time it was too hard to even hold a candle up, so in my hand, which was hanging at my side, I hung a lantern in my fingers.

'You don't need to hold it up, girl. Just keep it in your fingers.'

It was like the floodgates opened. I went to all kinds of dark places and just put light on myself in some form.

'All I need to do is remember the light,' I thought.

And this feeling of sacredness started filling me."

she kneeled at the cave entrance –
hands had quietly removed the snow and ice
that had blocked her view.
lit in warmth and sacredness
she gazed upon her cathedral.

"I'm wondering how many different moods we can hold at once? Is there a maximum number? Do we notice? Or do we just feel the dominant one? Or the dominant two?

Can we mix them together to work together?

What happens when happy dances with sad? Do they meld together and make something else? Can happy tap agitated on the shoulder and flip it over on top of sad? Will anger stand up or will contentment roll over and laugh?"

i commit to me, myself, today.
i vow to listen to and follow and believe in
my goodness.
to recognize my strength
and wield it with the added power of compassion.
to know my heart
and trust it and not turn to outside expectations
to feed it, but rather turn to my own inner guidance
to lead me.
to know that i am the woman i want to be
and work to uncover more of my beauty daily.
and to be gentle with myself when i slip –
loving myself even in the darkness.
to me, myself, i give my love.
and it is from me, myself, my love is returned.

"'Where's your identity? Where are your wells?' I asked myself that this morning.

If everything started changing for you, if you weren't sure of your health and what was ahead for you and your life, what would you do? What would you concentrate on? And I'm thinking the answer to that would be based on the answers to where's your identity, where are your wells?

Oh, in case you don't think like I do...by 'wells' I mean where do you go to fill yourself up?

I'm thinking this might be a good thing to figure out, and a good thing to adjust if the places aren't really that nourishing."

every question life could throw at her
swam in her head.
she had answers to nothing -
and she was lost.
all she had was what was inside of her.
she knew that was enough if she
could just let go and trust that.
if she could just let go and trust herself.
lifting one finger at a time,
she began to loosen her grip,
she began to let go.

"And so I sit and wonder. Who is it that we think we are? Who is it that we identify with inside of us? And do we get stuck there? If we're fluid-like and changing constantly, is it a deadly mistake to get stuck in one perspective? Which one am I stuck in? And how do I know when it's time to change? And why is it that it takes so much courage to change?"

at first she yanked them out slowly,
laying them in patterns.
feeling their importance.
now they weren't what mattered anymore.
it was getting thru that cloud that counted.
brushing the hooks off her arms,
scraping them off her body she gave them
little thought.
throwing them aside,
she gathered her self and headed for the
other side of the mist.

"All the problems I have, I can change. I have power over them. I don't have any horrible news coming my way that I can't change. If we have power over what's going on, how cool is that? Those are the easy problems! Even if they feel like the weight of the world.

Maybe they feel like the weight of the world exactly because we're NOT handling them. So let's get up and handle them. It's entirely up to us.

So that when the big tragic unchangeable news comes our way, and it comes in a thousand different forms to everyone, well, we'll know we didn't waste the good that we did have. Life is short! I so want to grab it!"

"missed opportunities" he said.
he had missed another.
how many had she missed,
she wondered.
it was up to her to grab the moments—
and she would.

"Sometimes when things run deep in me, they will act like filters to my thoughts. Every thought that runs through me will also run through that filter. I know it and watch it.

The filter these days is 'living.' Living fully, living with intention, living to uncover more of who I am. The preciousness of it all. The brevity of it all.

When I was thinking about a friend with marriage problems this morning, the thoughts ran through that filter. What I wish I could tell her more than anything is simple:

This is it.
This is your life.
Surround yourself with people who encourage you to be all you are, to be who you want to be. Even when it's different than who they are!

Step back.
Take a look at your life and what you're doing. Are you apologizing for who you are? Are you being less than who you are for someone else? If so, ask yourself why. And ask yourself what it is you gain with that choice.

Why would you choose to be with someone who doesn't encourage you and want you to be all of who you are?

It's such a simple concept. And yet, I'm not sure how easy it is to create.

It certainly has taken me a long time. And once you touch it, it doesn't mean you have it forever. It's a constant thing to work at. It can drift away in a moment. But I'm thinking that just the very process of demanding that in your life, and also giving that back in your life...I'm thinking the act of doing that is living fully.

It's like one big wonderful circle.

Are you living your life as you? Or are you living your life as your partner's perception of you?

It's one of those questions that you can like and hate all at once. It's a good one to get you thinking. It's one to hate because it causes more work. Hmm...I guess that's all the more reason to like it."

*you can try to feed the bear
but he will never get enough.
the best thing to do is feed yourself.*

"It was a gorgeous morning. And it was lost on me. I wore my hood for half of the walk, not paying much attention.

Woe.
I noticed what I was doing.
I realized I was distracted with something, I was feeling something.

Okay, what?

Discouraged. Yep. I was fully discouraged.

I took my hood off and looked at the sky. It's gorgeous. And I knew it. But it wasn't filling me up like it usually does. I watched that inside of me.

Do you close a door inside of you when you're discouraged? Or does the discouragement just take energy away? Probably both.

Do I try to change this mood? I have so much to do today and it's going to take energy. Do you actively work to change your mood or do you accept where you're at?

I came up with 'balance it.' Allow it to be, but don't wallow in it. Allow it to be, and allow it to leave when it's time for it to leave. Don't hang on to it. Don't encourage it. Just allow it.

I'm going to try to do that. It's a whole art I'm just beginning to notice. The art of allowing your emotions. I'm not real good at it yet. But I'm going to practice."

she'd been fighting herself so long now,
the idea of trusting herself seemed foreign.
and yet...if she could trust...
if she could just trust herself ~
she just might discover the best
friend she's ever known.

"Another muddle headed morning. My walk thoughts are scattered and harder to focus on.

In the middle of racing thoughts all over the place, I glanced over at the mountain of dirt that's in the construction site up the street.

It's huge. They've been building it up.

That mountain of dirt has been there for years now. They keep moving it around, changing the terrain a bit, and making it look different here and there. But it's always the same dirt.

As soon as I realized that, a shot of a thought went through me.

Same dirt.
Different mountain.

That's your struggles, Ter.

43

It's the same issues, same hang ups, same insecurities, same dirt – just shaped into different mountains throughout the years.

Wow.

That really affected me.

Okay, I said.

So what do I do with that???

Well, if it's the same stuff, just different emphasis at different times, you can probably learn from what works and what doesn't.

So what's not worked in the past?

Fear.

Right away fear comes to mind.
That hasn't worked.
Tightening up.
Grasping.
Clinging.
Closing down. (Although, that one's debatable, it has come in handy at times.)
Doubt.

Oh, doubt's a big one.
That never works.

What HAS worked?

Trust.
That darn stinking trust. That works.
Opening.
Knowing it's all okay.
Believing.
Gratitude. That works magic.

Okay.
Okay.

So.
You're looking at a mountain right now that's discouraging you. And you're doing all the things that don't work.

That's good, Terri, good planning there.
WHAT THE HECK ARE YOU DOING, GIRL?!

Why?
Why go to the things that don't work?

Because they're easier?
Noooo.
I mean, they are.
But not in the long run.
The wear and tear on the psyche isn't easier by any means.

Why do the wrong stuff?

I don't know...
Habits? Laziness? I just don't know.

But I do know I see it now. And I'm going to work on changing that. And I'm going to work on leveling the mountain.

When I'm old and getting ready to leave this world, I'd love to look at the terrain of my self and see that I leveled that mountain out, and built a field of flowers."

i want to stretch my soul way past anything
i've ever known.
i want to push my boundaries over the edge
and lose them forever.
i want to throw the limits away,
watching them shatter to dust.
i want to hold the darkness with ease
knowing it's an integral part of the light.
i want to fill with the calm knowing of trust,
and i want to love all the way to beyond.

"I think I figured out what old is.

Maybe old is when you stop learning and you tell yourself that's a good thing. When the comfortable ways are always the better ways and you have no desire to get out of your comfort zone, and you think that's an admirable way to be. You actually brag about that.

Maybe old is when people allow you to be that way and don't challenge you.

Woe.

Maybe that's the worst part. What is that saying when people don't even challenge you?

I just don't want to be old and telling people I have no interest in learning anything new. I want to learn to sculpt, and to throw clay, and play guitar, and sing and so many things.

But I'm thinking what I really need to do is relearn my reactions to life.

I'm thinking that's where my greatest challenges in life are. I'm thinking that if I wait until I'm eighty, I'm sunk. The time to start is today. So when I'm eighty, life won't be about being safe. It will be about being free. Life won't be about enduring. It will be about truly living."

unwrapping her hands
from around her heart,
she offered her all.

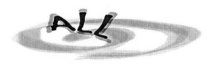

Magic.

I love that word. And I do think there's something to life that is magical. I do think when you touch certain things in a certain way, unexplained, marvelous things happen.

And I think gratitude is the key to having magic in your life. I have experienced it and know it. Seems I got lucky and was born with a lot of gratitude just flowing through me naturally. But I still lose it from time to time. And my gosh, when I do, it's as if someone took the colors out of life, the zest, the zip, the zing...all that 'z' stuff is gone. There's just a mid to low-level hum. Life becomes a drag.

It usually takes me awhile before I realize there's something missing. There's a feeling that something is 'off' and that things aren't zinging. And sooner or later, I figure it out. The gratitude left!

While I've gotten better at realizing the stuff is gone, I fumble when trying to figure out how to get it back. Different things work for different people. I cannot do the list of how much better off I am than someone in a third world country. That comes easy when I'm feeling the gratitude, but when I'm not, that generally makes me cranky. If you come to me and suggest that I do that, I may glare at you. I will think things like 'I am not stupid. I know I have everything in the world and compared to others I have no complaints. I know that. And I still feel bad. So there. Leave me alone.'

I need a different plan of action. Recently, I came up with a possibility for myself.

"I have these vague beliefs or thoughts or pieces of thoughts...things I just know in my heart. One is about gratitude. I believe it's as powerful as love. I need to repeat that. Gratitude is as powerful as love. It's overlooked a ton and I believe it's a force beyond our understanding.

Sometimes I watch when I don't have it. It's like I'm not alive. The zest is gone and I don't know how to get it back. But you know what? I never thought of this until now! The key may be in the the different angles of gratitude! There are different ways of looking at it. Something so big and powerful has got to have different angles.

So, it's not so simple as counting your blessings. Sometimes you're just not in a spot to do that. It doesn't have to be so elementary. That's where I've been, in gratitude elementary school. It's time to step up to gratitude middle school.

If you step up and to the side, tilt your head a little bit, squint over towards the sun...well then, maybe you can see whatever you're not feeling grateful about a little differently. And you can find something to honestly be grateful for. I think I could always do that if I didn't feel like I had to give a list of my blessings. Yeah, I think I could almost always find a little something to feel grateful for.

Like now. I'm not feeling totally grateful for my feeling of fear I'm having. Okay, okay, I'm not feeling grateful at all. And it has taken the zest out of things. But at the same time, there's a belief I have that I can hang on to. Actually there are several beliefs that I can hang on to! Beliefs like, I'll make it through this, and this fear won't last forever, and that the different angles approach is worth trying. And for THOSE beliefs and ideas, I can honestly feel grateful. They give me something to hold on to. They give me hope.

I'm not exactly grateful for the ditch or for falling into the darn ditch. And I'm not exactly grateful for all the effort it will take to pull myself up on this rope out of the darn ditch.

But the rope! The rope of hope? Oh, yes! For THAT I'm grateful.

There's always got to be something to hold. Even if it's just a tiny seed. And maybe that's all I need to find sometimes. Now, will I always WANT to find it? No. But that's my choice, isn't it? I can choose to put the effort into making my life magically zestful or I can choose to be a zombie at times. The choice is mine. And at least now, I have a way I can try to work with that choice."

I think recognizing that we don't always want gratitude is really big. That goes with any of my emotions. Sometimes I want to feel angry or hopeless or frustrated. I can't exactly figure out why. Laziness, self indulgence - many not so good reasons come to mind. And I don't think it's a good choice on my part. But I do think that recognizing the fact that I am making that choice, no matter how lame, matters.

Once I know the choice is up to me, I can decide where to go from there. Am I going to frustrate myself and make myself crazy by trying to find that darn stupid rope of hope... or am I going to admit I just want to wallow for a bit? And then allow myself wallowing time? Or am I going to recognize I'm wallowing, and really want better for myself, and turn myself around and look for that incredible rope called hope? It is in those moments when I'm trying to figure out where it is I really want to go that I stand before my power. I need to recognize that and acknowledge that.

"I know this for a fact, if I focus on the gratitude and see the good, I can change my mood around. I know that. I believe that. Inside though, is this powerful force that's angry and frustrated and tired and grouchy. Gratitude just doesn't look appealing to that force. Whatever is going on is strong. It's big to me. And it's important to me. My insides want to head to the negative full steam ahead.

I am standing at an important place.

Not even so much because of the outcome of the 'situation.' But because of the broader picture, because of the choice I make inside myself for my life goal. I know what I've got to do. And at this point, I don't want to. I just don't want to. I'm going to spend the next few hours trying to get to a spot where I can go to the gratitude.

Because I know that's the direction I REALLY want to go. I just know the other direction is way easier.

The phrase 'follow your heart' comes to mind. I like that phrase and believe in it. Thing is...you have to hear the whole thing. If I followed what was on top of my heart, it'd be a whole different kind of thing than if I follow what's way, way down deep. You have to hear the whole thing.

And then you have to have the courage to follow it."

finding the crack of light,
she pried her fingers in its edges.
pulling the darkness back
with all her strength,
the ocean of light poured forth.
weeping tears of gratitude,
she felt the Light flood over her.

49

I found a blog entry that I had written when I was really struggling and feeling overwhelmed. I smiled when I saw how I ended the thoughts.

"For all those who think I'm courageous,
I'm not.
I don't have the courage right now.
I really don't.

Sometimes the stuffing just gets knocked right outta me.

But I'm going to try anyway.
Because I've come way too far to take the easy way out now.

Thing is...
I get confused on what's right and what's not.

And then it occurs to me, gratitude is never wrong, is it?
Should be a pretty safe place to start."

Maybe sometimes when we're struggling, it's hard to find the gratitude. But maybe at other times, having gratitude isn't really the problem. It's other stuff that's throwing us off. Maybe we're low on courage or trust. And maybe starting in a place of gratitude is the magic we need to find those other things.

she closed her eyes
and thought of her year.
it couldn't be just the "good" she was
thankful for.
it had to be the "all"...
the fullness, the depths, the journey.
the dance of Life.
for these she gave thanks.

"Maybe it's delicious even when it isn't.

I like that sentence.

Today wasn't exactly delicious. It was more 'challenging' than anything else. But the delicious part that I found just now? It was that I made it through and knew all along that I had a choice of what I was going to chose to grab and hold on to.

I think just knowing that there is a choice actually helps you choose the better thing to hold.

Maybe the delicious doesn't go away.
Maybe we do.
Maybe it's always delicious.
Maybe sometimes you just have to see it through, stick around, and maybe peek under a few layers of crust to find the good stuff, all the while knowing the delicious is in there somewhere."

I find it really hard to find any kind of delicious when I'm dealing with loss. I think so much of my struggle is because I want things to be a certain way, and I want things to last forever. And I don't hold the most basic truth about life...that it's changing all the time. In struggling with it on one of my walks, I had the following conversation with myself.

"Love and loss are part of the same coin. To excel at one, you must excel at the other. Life is loss. It's constant change. People are here on their own journeys. They come and they go. Some come in and stay a long time. Some leave in a huff. Some leave quietly and sadly. Some hang on way after it's time for them to leave.

It's all about change.
Change.
Change.
Change.

It's not about staying the same. It's not about forever. It's not. That entire perspective must be turned upside down if I'm ever going to really grasp living. If the goal is to become love, or to uncover the love inside of me, then part of the goal MUST be to accept loss.

And so I thought of accepting loss. I get all caught up in the feelings and compassion and letting go gets even harder. If it's accepting loss do I turn into some kind of non-compassionate person who doesn't feel anything?

No.

Each loss must change me in some way. It must. Because if loss and love are part of the same coin, then that coin changes you every time it's part of your life. It's the nature of the coin. And those changes are the deep, quiet ones you can't really tell people about. But they're the ones that put lines on your face, and a certain look in your eyes. Those are the things that will turn you into that wise old crone. If you let them.

Loss doesn't have to take away from you. It can most certainly add to who you are. A loss doesn't have to leave a hole. It can add a light, a spark, a knowing. And it can leave holes too. But the holes aren't pointless pain things. They matter. They're okay. Even if they do hurt.

If I'm ever going to get this 'living love' stuff down, I have got to change some very major perspectives here. I have got to not only accept loss, I have to embrace loss as much as I embrace love, for then I am embracing all of life.

And that fear of pain that freaks me out with loss now?
That entire perspective must also change. Pain isn't a killer. Fear is.

Fear is.

And then my mind rolled back to the moments I have, how short it all is even if I do live to an old age. Grabbing the moments, living in the present, dropping the fear, embracing loss, embracing change, and knowing THAT is living.

Woe.

I guess I'm going to get some practice here. And maybe THAT'S how I can honor those I love and have lost – by getting this lesson."

"it's not so much the hole inside me
that i mind," she said.
"it's the weight that's in that hole."
"then take the weight out and
leave it behind and fill the hole
with things that will make you fly,"
was her reply.

it is your tears that run down your face,
and yet i taste their salt.
it is your hand that wipes your cheek,
and yet i feel the softness of your skin.
when you turn to face your world,
you never leave me.
you are part of me.
i am with you.

Recently, a friend called me, sobbing. She had lost a love in her life and was devastated. It was hard to try to just be there for her knowing I couldn't do anything to change what was going on. She passionately proclaimed she'd never love anyone again. It hurt too much. I heard her voice and wondered. I knew the feeling, and I didn't want to discount it. It is so strong and so true at that moment. I hoped for her though, that it wouldn't stay true.

Her call reminded me of a call I had gotten years before. Someone I just barely knew, but who was very familiar with my bone sighs, called me one night out of the blue. She had experienced a major trauma and needed to talk to someone. The bone sighs had touched her, and she thought of me and called. I remember very clearly hanging up after a long conversation. I was so filled with compassion and complete confusion as to what in the world she would do now after such an experience. It was that night I wrote the bone sigh called 'splinters.'

*she built her cathedral
from the splinters of
her shattering.*

That's all we can do, I thought as I hung up after this most recent phone call.

"We rebuild. Over and over again. We rebuild. And if we're aware, we do way more than rebuild. We build our cathedrals."

I feel fortunate that these women called me to share their pain. Both of them were in agony, and both trusted their hearts with me. Each time I truly wanted to just fix it for them, take it away, say something so profound that they would feel healed, and all the while I knew, there was absolutely nothing I could do but listen.

"I kept on thinking. I thought about the pain involved and how it does something to us and changes us and drops walls at the same time it puts walls up. There are connections that are so incredibly real and raw through pain. The walls drop at certain moments and we see each others' souls. It's such a weird, weird thing. It's horrible to have the pain, and yet, it's real. And there's a closeness there. We all have trauma. And the touching of souls that can happen when we share it is incredible. What a mix living is, what an amazing mix."

holding you close,
my heart whispered to yours,
"i'll help you thru this.
i am with you.
you are not alone."

there was talking and noise
and people trying to help.
i sat quietly reading every inch of your face -
desperately looking for a way
to take this from you.
all i could find were ways to share
it with you.
walking next to you, we'll go forward.

I've been through my own stuff, and some of it seemed pretty black. And it was. But I discovered a blackness of a different kind when I walked through a suicide in my family. I thought I had experienced an earthquake in my life before, but never had I experienced anything like this. I tried to be present for my family, and be by their sides as they walked through the grief that had come slamming down on top of them. The helplessness I felt and still feel can be overwhelming. I taped up the word 'acceptance' over my desk for about a year, trying to get some part of the meaning of the word into my life. After a year, I figured it wasn't working, and maybe I needed to try another word. I took 'acceptance' down one day, and in total defiance, threw it in the trash can.

Deep down I think that's the correct word, it's the word that I need, the concept that I need. I just don't think it's an easy one to get or to keep at all. And I wonder about the ones who were so completely devastated by that loss, do they ever find acceptance in what happened? I really don't know. I can't imagine that. I like to hope for it, but I can't imagine it.

> "I discovered something one day. Actually, I heard it come out of my mouth one night when I was talking to someone who was hurting about as much as you can hurt. I heard myself tell him that it wasn't all black - that I had figured it out - that I had thought that it was, but that it wasn't. And I heard myself talk about the power of love and caring between people. And how I had never seen darkness so black before, but even in that blackness, I saw tiny spots of light in the love I felt for him.
>
> As I spoke, I listened to my words. I realized while it was the closest thing to Hell I had ever been involved in, it wasn't Hell.
>
> 'Hell is not love anymore.'
> Someone famous once said that, I think. That's not mine. I sure like that line. And if you have anyone reaching out to you in the darkness, even if they have nothing else they can do but put their hand out and stretch their fingers your way, those very fingers give off light.
>
> Hell is not love anymore.
> I have never ever come close to that.
> And I hope I never do.
> Light.
> It's all around us.
> If we look.
> Sometimes just tiny spots of light.
> But they're there. They're so there. Hang on to them.
> Never let them go."

*the solitary flight
brings unimagined strength
and opens the heavens.*

The dance we do with standing up on our own and facing things alone and leaning on each other, and needing each other is such an intricate one. As with most things in my life, it seems to make sense when I view it in layers. I need people and I want to need them (mostly). At the same time, I really believe this journey is ours to go alone. That the growing and the stretching and the becoming more is up to us alone.

"There's a thought lodged in my brain. It won't get out. It won't move. I guess that's because I haven't had much of a chance to really sit with it. The thought...the question...is...

What if you really understand that it's yours to go alone? What if you really accept that and are okay with that? Where does that leave you?

Seems to me it would have to leave you in one heck of a good spot. A spot where you put less pressure on the things and people around you. The fact that they are there through part of the journey rocks. And that's it. There doesn't have to be any more than that. They don't need to do anything. Or be anything. Or offer anything. Expectations slow down. The lonely feeling would slow down because you would already know that you are alone and anything extra is gravy. Gratitude would pick up. Seems like it'd be a good thing all around.

And I feel like I'm just now seeing this really clearly. I must have seen this before. Maybe? But with me, it's waves. Things come in clear, I get them. Then whoosh! They wash away and I forget I ever saw them. Or there's just a vague memory left.

This is one heck of a cool wave. Wonder how long I can ride it.

Alone.

Riding the wave alone. And loving it."

it was the nature of the game –
while the love was there surrounding him,
the work was his alone.
the journey would be solitary
and the flight extraordinary.

59

it is in your solo flight that your
wings become filled with power,
the clouds part,
and the heavens open.

I get pretty excited about these thoughts, type them out on my blog or talk to my friends about them. And sometimes I forget that they really may only make sense in my own mind, that maybe the way I'm phrasing something sounds pretty strange to someone else, and I can cause them to worry about me! That happened with this concept as I sat across the table from a girlfriend of mine. She looked concerned as I excitedly told her I wanted to live my life on my own. I think she thought I was operating from a place of hurt and fear and was closing people out. Not so at all. But totally understandable that she would think that. And so, I found myself typing yet another blog after having tea with her.

"I talked to a friend yesterday about being on the journey alone and she hesitated because at first she thought that I was talking about not needing people, not leaning on people. Closing myself off from people.

Oh my, no.

I need people. And leaning is something I know how to do well. But there's a big difference between needing help and support from your friends and needing things that only you can give yourself.

THAT'S the journey alone - giving yourself the things that can only come from inside of you.

I think I've slipped there. I think I've been looking for things other people can't give me. What's that about? And why? That seems to be the killer of any relationship, any kind of relationship.

Bam.
Kill.
Zap.

Why would I do that?
Is it because I get lazy?
Or do I just not see straight when I get comfortable?

I don't know what it is. But there's no good reason for it. And you might as well give your relationships away if you go in that direction, Ter. You might as well give yourself away. Because that's what you're doing. You're kind of messing up everyone's power when you go in that direction.

I see this as a real chance to get back on track. A reach chance to see who I am and work with myself.

I remember once having this thought: what if I treated my inner self like I treat my best girlfriend?

I pictured my friend coming into my kitchen and how I listen with interest with all she has to say and how I support her so easily. What if I did that with myself?

Well, all this alone journey talk - it's not alone.
IT'S WITH ME!
My best girlfriend!
What if I actively, with awareness and presence, traveled with myself?

And what if I was really comfortable with that and allowed everyone else to pop in as they wished, when they wanted to. My gosh. I love this idea."

alone.
surrounded by love
and yet totally alone,
the victory is up to you.
and the power is gained
in that solitary flight.

PROTECTING
YOUR
vulnerabilities

pushing hard against the walls,
she broke thru into a sea of vulnerability.
it's where she knew she had to be
if she was going to honestly know love.

Ohmygosh. Vulnerabilities. It is so hard to be vulnerable. Actually, I take that back. I'm pretty good at being vulnerable to a point. I put my thoughts out, I share, I open my heart. But the stuff that's really down deep, that only a very few people have the power to touch...oh that stuff...that stuff can make or break a person.

But that's the thing we just have to do – open our hearts, even the vulnerable spots. That's what I truly believe will bring us to another place. That's what will open the door for us to become love.

For me, the bone sigh that hits the hardest is the following:

strength lies in the opening of the heart.

It seems like such a simple sentence. Oh yeah, you have to be strong to be open. Are you kidding me??? We're talking being like Hercules here. Some of the times that require the most effort on my part are with the people I love and trust the most. I guess because they have the most power to really hurt. Those very people know my weak spots, know my buttons, and know my patterns. They also equally have the power to help me grow.

> "Being vulnerable isn't my favorite feeling in the world. But when it's held with kindness and love...THAT is something I have no words for."

you have taught me the strength of tenderness.

63

"My heart got so broken open.
My heart.
It wasn't my body or my bank. It was my heart.

Of course.
It had to have been.

I just nodded.

I NEEDED my heart to be broken open so that I could – ohmygosh – I
don't know what...

Rebuild it?
Refill it?
Put it back together with my own love?
Learn self love?

I don't know...but I so know I needed it.
Wow. Wow. Wow. Go figure.

For a long time I've known it was a good thing. That I got a lot of good out
of it. But I'm not sure I knew that I NEEDED it!

My heart. Go figure.
Me and my heart. We needed to break a bit.
I have to remember that when I try so hard to protect it."

~~~~~

"I'm stuck on my vulnerabilities, my hurts. Stuck on me. But if I look on
over at the other person and see that I trust their basic intentions (and I
may have to work with that and look deeper than whatever it is that has
happened to hurt me)...if there's a basic trust in their intentions towards
me, then I need to keep my eyes on that.

If I keep my eyes there, I can go and work it out. If I keep my eyes on me,
then I get stuck and shut down. It's a trust issue...and how deep the trust
goes...and keeping your eyes on the trust, not the doubt. A question of
where you put your emphasis...where you put your power.

Wow. If I could just live all this stuff..."

the past rose up with incredible strength
pulling me away.
opening my eyes,
i focused on your face
and whispered thru tears 'i choose you.'
and the past faded away.

do you need this protection?
will it serve your highest good?
or will it stunt you and disconnect you
and leave you empty?
time to decide.
grab your trust,
squash the fear,
and kick your way thru that wall.
you've got a better place to head to.

Ah, and if I can even get close to where it is I want to go there will be deep changes inside me. I will understand that others really cannot hurt me. That all of that is inside of me, and up to me.

> maybe being love is knowing you've okay –
> that they can't hurt you...
> knowing the power to hurt you is yours alone.
> then maybe being love is using your power
> to offer compassion.
> all they while knowing they've okay too.

It's the looking within to really learn how to love that will expand me. I'm just beginning to really see how it might work.

"...But that's the easy love.

That's the love that comes naturally, flows easily, fits in with my dance steps, and moves with me. Easy Peasy.

But what about the love that doesn't do that? The love that's challenging. The love that means if you can pull it off, you're really pulling it off. That love.

The stuff that requires you to see people for who they are and accept all of that - even when parts of it hurt.

The part that requires you to look at yourself and to see and understand your reactions, and get beyond them, step around them, and give love back even when it feels funky.

The part about giving love back to get nothing in return.

To just give it.
To honestly, honestly just give it.
The part that requires bone deep acceptance.

The part that requires faith and a knowing and a belief that it's all okay just as it is.

The part that requires trust beyond any trust you've ever given.

The part that requires giving beyond any giving you've ever known.

The love that demands you to be all of who you are.

THAT stuff.

THAT stuff is what I'm just learning. That's where I'm in kindergarten."

the flood was knocking and she knew it.
opening the door, she released her grasp
and stepped aside.
the trickle flowed in slowly at first.
then stronger and stronger
the current picked up.
pulling her under,
carrying her with it, she lost herself
and became the water.

now you'll learn to have a true loving relationship.
and it will bring you to your knees,
knock you down over and over again.
but if you master it, girl...
you will have learned what you asked for.
if you only have the strength to love
beyond yourself,
you will find the answers.

"Well, I'm thinking now's the time for foolhardy. Only the foolhardy can touch love like I want to touch love. Only the foolhardy can live like I want to live. This fear stuff sucks. Enough already. One. Two. Three. LEAP!"

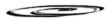

"Loving someone completely, being vulnerable and trusting and open... those things just don't happen. It's not just chemistry. It's work and it's scary and it's decisions and choices and it's a journey. And there is no way on earth it's a part-way thing. I think there's a rule somewhere. Journeys of a life time can't be part way things. And I'm kind of glad about that. Because I think I'd be chicken enough to only go part way if they were! As it is, I'm in for the whole deal. The whole shabang. Learning how to be whole and loving whole – all the way to beyond."

i want to enter your sacred ground,
to hold you in the depth of your spirit,
to be surrounded by the mists of your soul
and to soak in the essence of you.
it's a giving and a taking i honor quietly,
solemnly.
if your door is open,
i am there.

But what about the unhealthy stuff? The stuff we find ourselves trapped in. Sometimes we never leave those traps. And sometimes, we may have left it physically, but it is still holding us down. It's still such a part of where we're operating from. What do we do with that stuff?

She had been drinking that night. I called to check in on her. She was walking through darkness and I knew it. We had talked a lot and I had just tried to hold her with my words. This night though, there was too much to even try to hold. She was pouring it out and the pain was soaking me, drenching me. I sat there wondering what I could possibly offer to relieve her agony. I listened, held her in my heart and tried to let her know I understood. I tried to help her and knew that she couldn't hear me. When I got off the phone I didn't know what to do with all she had just handed me. And so I wrote.

for women everywhere

something snapped inside of her.
'ENOUGH ALREADY' she screamed.
it's time for women everywhere to claim their worth,
their value, their beauty, their sacredness.
no more of this believing the darkness
that's been thrust upon them.
no more taking the blame for the sins of others.
no more claiming themselves failures
when in fact, they are survivors.
it's time for women to stop.
turn around.
face those people who have hurt,
harmed and wounded
and let them know that they refuse to be destroyed.
they refuse to carry the burden.
it's time for women everywhere to place the palms of
their hands on their wounds,
acknowledge the pain
and change the world with
the lessons gained from that pain.
it's time to move with the wisdom
of a survivor and to know your strength.
the world is waiting for us.
let us step up now and reclaim ourselves,
and reclaim the world.

Women are survivors. Maybe all people are but women are the ones I talk intimately with. They are the ones who share their stories with me. They are the ones who tell me of the hell that they have experienced and they are the ones I watch get up and move forward. Sometimes I am overwhelmed with the strength I witness, with the story that has led these women to their own awareness of their power and their beauty. Sometimes my heart breaks as I watch women miss that part, moving forward in vain. We need to see ourselves. We need to help each other see. Not all women make it. We need to reach out to each other and pull each other along. We need to help each other survive.

she wept
and she ached
and she held her head.
they had died because
they had never been seen.
she felt an iron determination creep over her.
it was time to see herself –
and honor them.

Seeing them. Seeing ourselves. Knowing we are valuable and acting upon that knowing. I think sometimes it takes changing a whole lifetime of lessons we were taught. Just trying to navigate through life acting like you count can be a complete whirlwind of confusion. How do you balance taking care of others and taking care of you?

she wasn't them.
she couldn't be.
was she going to claim
herself as herself or
forever be halfway between worlds?

"How should a person interact with unhealthy love in a loving way? What does one do with the other people - the ones with the unhealthy needs who feel unloved unless those needs are met? Where does that kind of thing leave you? That is one heck of a question isn't it? I see it all around me with friends and their lives, me and my life, and people I hear about. I believe it's everywhere. We all have this question to face.

I'm thinking the answer's got to be about ourselves. It's got to be about who we are. Everything we do has got to be with the purpose of honoring who we are. With that in mind, the oddest answer for myself surfaces.

I must speak my truth in every situation.
Hmmm. Could it be that easy?

Can I say something like 'I feel funny about this. It doesn't feel like love to me and I want to offer love. This other way is the way it feels right to me, so I want to let you know that this is what I'll do. And I want you to know that to me, this is loving you.'

Oh wow. Could I ever get that clear and straight? I can actually see doing that in some situations and having it work. And then, in others, I can see their reactions to that being closing down and shutting me out. But then again, maybe that's okay. Maybe that's not my choice.

Maybe the only choice I can make is offering my truth. And then letting everyone else make their own choice based on that.

How totally empowering to do my best to offer what I feel is healthy and let everyone chose if they want it or not. And then for me to be okay with their choices.

That would be strength.
That would be integrity.
That would be awesome."

they won't always reach back, she said.
know, tho, that there are those who will.
love them. honor the others.
and believe in what it is you are offering.

71

*after all,
she did allow it, didn't she?
if she allowed it,
did she believe they were right?
time to face her beliefs honestly.
and her responsibility to herself.*

"I just found myself in a situation that required my giving of myself. This has prompted me to think about the whole concept of giving this morning. There's quite a range of 'receivers' out there to give to. I've got people in my life who are just so grateful for things you do for them, they can't thank you enough. I've got people who I believe are grateful but they just can't say much about it. I've got people who don't even notice. And I've got people who never quite get enough or it's never quite given in a good enough way; something is always wrong.

I thought of that this morning.

I'm a people pleaser. I try real hard to please. Long stories with that...

I try to watch things now. Make sure I'm doing what I'm doing for healthy reasons. Not to try to please the planet like I used to. To make sure I don't throw me away in the process of pleasing.

I think a whole lot of women (people) deal with that one.

So I caught myself wanting to go back to the giving I just did and tweak it a bit. Make it better. Make it something more of what they wanted.

Um.
Stop.
Hello??

What is it they really want, Ter?

And I realized that what they really, really wanted, I honestly could not give.

All I could give was what I offered.

And so I resisted the tug I was feeling.

What was it I REALLY wanted?

What was REALLY causing the tug?

Was it because I gave wrong?
Was it because it was perceived wrong?
Was it because I just really wished they'd see me and accept me?

Um.
Yes. That was it. The last choice there.

And there we find some pretty deep roots of this people pleaser.

The thing is, I've dealt with those roots a lot. Untwisted them, untangled them, looked at them, snipped some of them. I know them very, very well by now.

And so I sat back and thought about giving.

When you give, Ter, it has to be for YOUR reasons. And it has to be for your highest good. What is the reason you are giving? Is it to give or is it to get? Don't give to get. That just doesn't work on so many levels. Give to give. Give what you can. And let it be.

It's then up to the receiver to do what they will with the gift.

And it is a gift.

Perhaps the receiver will never know that if you, yourself, don't know it."

maybe when you really love yourself
you can see beyond that self -
and then maybe you never give yourself away.
maybe you just give.

73

To see yourself - to see beyond yourself - you can't hide who you are.

"Do not hide who you are for anyone's sake."

That was a sentence I found in one of my blogs. I don't know what the blog was about. I just snipped the sentence out and put it in my folder here. As I sat holding it in my hands, I had a memory that made me sad.

When I was in my early twenties, I left the Catholic Church. It was a difficult decision for me as I was raised Catholic and had considered myself a devout Catholic for a long time. I knew that it would affect my parents, I felt pressure to stay, but it was something I had to do.

After telling my parents, my father asked me to keep that decision hidden from my grandparents. His request weighed heavily on me for many different reasons. And now, as a woman in her late forties, I can tell you, I would never even consider doing it. But at the time, in my early twenties, against my heart, I did what he asked.

It changed my entire relationship with my grandparents. I went from feeling close to them to feeling uncomfortable and false. After my grandmother died, I had numerous nightmares about my relationship with her. It has been something that truly has haunted me.

Who I was then was not someone to be ashamed of. I believe my father felt it would reflect poorly on him and he didn't want that.

If someone thinks that who you are when you follow your heart is someone who makes them look bad, then perhaps there needs to be some examining of what is happening.

It's an area that my father and I never examined together, and now it is something that I regret. At the same time, I learned something powerful there. I will never again hide who I am for anyone's sake. And if anyone feels this is a problem in their life, I see this as their issue and not my own. It is not something I ever want to hold for someone again. They can hold it. Not me.

some believed in her.
others did not.
she joined the circle of believers
and rejoiced with them.

As I turned back to my folder that held all kinds of snippets from my blogs, I found another short little one that made me gasp.

"To see, you have to allow yourself to be seen."

Woe. Once again I have no idea what I was talking about or what that was from. But my gosh, it sure seems to tie into the theme here. I wonder what I meant when I wrote that. I sit here and think about my story with my grandparents. Maybe it's about seeing myself. If I could really see myself then, and really know my beauty and my value, I would have allowed myself to be seen by everyone. I would not have bowed to a request that did not honor that seeing.

Maybe when you don't allow yourself to be seen, you are ignoring who you are. Not only are others not seeing you, but neither are you. I worked really hard for years on the concept of seeing myself. I struggled over that for so long, maybe because I had gotten so good at hiding myself. Maybe those two things are directly connected.

> the power lie in the seeing.
> until she could see herself
> with her own eyes,
> she would not regain her power.

And yet, that's all about seeing yourself, but how about seeing others? I have found that for others to share themselves with me, I have to step forward and share myself with them. When I offer who I am, and allow hidden parts of me to show, then something happens. There's a vulnerability there - they feel it, seem to honor it, and then offer parts of themselves to me. It happens frequently. Enough for me to be a believer in it. And so, I step up and show myself and ask gently 'will you show me you too?' And then, to honor their response, I have to remember to really look.

> needing to feel safe
> she had labeled him
> and put him in a box.
> soon she found she needed honesty
> more than safety.
> she removed the box
> and found him grinning.

"One of the wild flowers that is abundant around here this time of year is the Tickseed Sunflower. It's this perky yellow flower that lines the sides of the roads. I absolutely love these flowers. They're growing in bunches up at one of the construction sites and they were so pretty this morning I just had to stop and look at them.

'Wow. If I were a flower I wouldn't mind being one of them,' I thought. And that's all it took. My mind was off and running with flowers and which ones I'd be.

'I wouldn't be a rose,' I thought. That seems like so much work. Now, I love roses, and think they're gorgeous. But I'm just not a rose.

Hmmm...that got me thinking.
Why is it too much work to be a rose? Roses don't work at being roses. They just are.

Okay, how about lilies and iris? Oh, yeah, too much work. For me. Not if you're a lily or an iris. Then it's easy.

Daisies and buttercups? Easy. I'd be them.

Chicory. That's me.

As silly as it sounds, the flower deal here gave me this great understanding of being comfortable with who I am.

There have been times in my life I had wished I could be gorgeous for a day. Or glamorous or worldly elegant. You know, just for a little bit. Some of those moments came back to me as I walked. I grinned at the thought of a rose being too much work.

A rose to me symbolizes the gorgeous or glamorous or worldly elegant.

I just ain't ever gonna be no rose.

But when I put all the flowers in front of my mind, there was none that was 'less than.' Each one was gorgeous in its own way.

And while this sounds like a silly story you'd tell an eight year old, it made sense to me. Maybe to my inner eight year old.

And I knew that being what came naturally to me was what I wanted to be. And that it didn't matter who was chicory and who was an iris and who was a buttercup. We all rock the world with our different colors.

I had not been struggling with my own image lately, it hadn't been a current issue, hadn't been on my mind. But this odd sense of understanding sunk into this ol' head of mine today. And this incredible sense of comfort in my own self covered me.

And the best part was that I realized I wasn't just one flower. The flower I was at any moment depended on my mood, the day, what was going on. Because no one is just one flower. Everyone's a bouquet."

lifting the cover of shame and self doubt,
she dropped it on the ground.
stepping into the light,
she slowly lifted her head.
this is who i am.
and i am here.
and i am enough.
the light warmed her face
and her heart.

Is there anything more wonderful than the love women share with their friends? As I grow older, the brilliant treasure of the friendships I hold shines brighter and brighter. When I was at my lowest point in life, the people I really trusted were my closest friends. I truly feel like they saved my life. I've heard that same sentiment from other women, and I nod knowingly each time I hear it.

as she thought of her friend,
she recalled hearing that
"gratitude is the heart of prayer."
she smiled, realizing her entire being
was one big prayer at that moment.
and her friend the reason for that prayer.

" - An offering to someone I love – An offering to everyone I love -

We talked yesterday. And earlier today. You told me you were confused about who you were. I sit here kind of confused on some stuff myself. Not so much of who I am. I don't think so, anyway...maybe though. I don't know.

Maybe it's more of what I believe in. Maybe it's more of why there's so much sadness so many times. I tell myself I know the answer to that one. I don't know though.

I read recently that 'life is struggle.' Man, they aren't kiddin', are they? The book also said if we could get comfortable with that idea, it'd be a lot easier.

Sometimes I think I have it. Sometimes I think I'm comfortable with it. And then I hear something like the struggle in your voice, and I know I'm just kidding myself. I'm not comfortable at all. I want to help. I want to fix it. I want to take it from you. I want to help you figure it out. I want to walk through it with you. And while you know I'll be boppin' around the edges – I can only go so deep.

That feels weird to me. Sometimes I don't think anyone's ever been deeper in me than you. And I feel like I've been pretty far inside of you too. And yet, it's still only the edges I can reach to try to help you.

I can listen to your stories of your past stuff. I can remember some of the details you've told me. I can try to help you sort through all of that. And I know all of that has brought you to where you are now. To who you are now.

All I know is who you are now. And who you've been throughout our friendship. That's the person I know, and that's the person I love. And that is the person I can remind you of. That is the person you're getting confused on. And I can help you there.

I see a woman who's made it through so much. Who's traveled so far. Who's grown so incredibly tall and strong and yet, who needs to be able to bend and lean. A woman filled with wisdom and love and heart. A woman who can touch me so deeply just by being herself. A friend who teaches me life, who teaches me about myself. A friend who has cracked my heart wide open and taught me how to love deeper. A woman who has changed my life. A friend who's hand I hold always. Always.

When you doubt it, when you don't know it, think of that. Remember how much I love you. And hold that.

You know I don't have any of this God stuff down. You know I can't figure any of it out. But my gosh, I know there's something to the idea that love is God. The depth of caring, the depth of love, that's somehow tangled up in God stuff. And that's what I want to throw your way now that it sounds like you need a life preserver.

A tangled up mess of Goddish love stuff. Figures, huh?
All I've ever had to offer you was a tangled up mess of stuff. Picture it. A tangled up mess of woven-sloppy-interlaced-God-love-me-friendship-you-us-our history-our future-trust-the universe-life preserver.

Hold it. Just plain ol' hold it. Don't let it go. I'm on the other end."

who do i thank for her?
the stars?
the universe?
she herself?
none of these thanks seem enough for
such a gift as having her in my life.

"There is nothing wrong with you, my friend. You call and ask me with that desperate tone that hurts to hear, and I'm sure must hurt to house.

You are beauty walking around that doesn't know it. You are strength and goodness and heart. And yeah, I know – you are darkness and anger and craze and passion. You are yin and yang, my friend.

Sometimes these opposites flow so smoothly and then sometimes they churn inside you. I think when the churning starts, the self doubt rises and bubbles and you start to feel like you're drowning.

You're not drowning. You may go under, you may get bumped around in the whirlpool, but you'll come up again. And you'll flow again.

The trick, I think, is to know that. To know that it's all a cycle. It's all a flow. Sometimes smooth, sometimes not.

The rope of trust is there for you. And now seems like the time when you need it. Hold on to it, and pull yourself up when you need that air. Trust in the process. Trust in your growth. Trust in who you are. And if you can't find the rope - look over in my eyes. There's one inside me just for you. We'll pull together."

it is in your struggle i see your spirit.
it is to your spirit
i give my heart.

Yes, I think every single one of us is spectacular. My word of choice is 'magnificent.' I think each one of us magnificent. And yet I found myself writing a note yesterday that said none of us were spectacular. What I meant is that if you wait for that feeling of being spectacular to do something with what's inside of you, you may never do anything.

I had gotten into a conversation with a young woman I have come to care a lot about. Her writing and her words touch me deeply. This young woman is also a cutter. She cuts herself to deal with the pain in her life. I asked her if together we could find a creative outlet where she could channel those feelings, and maybe use that in place of cutting. I suggested her writing and that maybe she could offer that to the world. She said she didn't feel spectacular enough in any particular thing to offer it anywhere. I wrote her the following note. I share it here for anyone who experiences similar feelings.

"here's the deal.
do with it what you will.

none of us are spectacular.
no one.
we're all the same.
 and we're all unique.

it's like a ton of different slants on the same thing.
our humanness.

some take their slant and never think it's worth anything.
some take their slant and claim it's worth more than others'.
some take their slant and feed their ego.
some take their slant and use it for a crutch.
some take their slant and offer it to the world in hopes it will help
someone else. there's a million ways we take what's inside of us and do
something/nothing with it.

you have experienced pain that others experience.
you can take it and use it to better the world.
or not. it's really your choice.

believing that offering what we have inside of us betters the world is a
belief i have now. but i had to learn it. i didn't know it until i did it.

i can't expect you to just believe me and just know what i'm saying is true.
you do have a choice to find out for yourself though.

and i think those are the things you have to ask yourself.

and if that's not what you are interested in now, what is it that you are
interested in? and why?

those questions matter. only you can ask them. only you can answer them.
only you can live them.

it's our lives.
what we do with them is up to us.
ya know?"

I didn't hear back from her for a few days. And then I went to her blog. One of the blogs she follows had a post on beauty. In that post, the blogger asked others to write their own thoughts on beauty in their own blogs. My friend had started and began talking of her feelings on the subject. After a few thoughts, she took a turn - straight into announcing to the world that she was a cutter. The tears poured down my cheeks as I read her post. She explained why she did what she did, and for the first time ever, I understood it. It's always been something that I couldn't wrap my head around. I saw her putting all of herself out there, knowing that friends and family would read her words. And I was so proud of her courage.

One of the gifts I got with bone sigh arts is that I get to hear from all sorts of different people about what they're going through. The people who relate to bone sighs have had pain in their lives that the bone sighs speak to. They write and share their stories. I've read enough of these now, and have watched enough people progress over the years that I've discovered something.

The people who take their pain and do something with it for someone else seem to gather some sense of healing. Reaching out and offering is part of the healing process. I believe that. It doesn't have to be on some big world wide scale, it can be right in our own little corner. Wherever it is, when it's offered from the heart, it does something. I am convinced. Those who don't reach out and turn inward and grow their world smaller, seem to suffer more. The healing seems to get stunted. It has been fascinating for me to watch.

This young woman did it with her blog. She reached out and put herself out there. I want to gather every cutter there is and point them in her direction. I sit back and smile at the controlling side of myself and let it go. I know the people who need her will find her, because she took her first step towards them.

throwing the limits away,
she watched them shatter to dust.

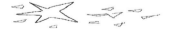

82

"The power and impact of each person is staggering. The blindness we all have towards that is equally as staggering. If we knew - if we really knew it - understood it, and believed it...would we do anything differently???"

~~~~~

"The power our acts have over other people is astounding. I need to brand that on my heart and hold that with all the respect it deserves."

Over and over I see the influence we have on each other, and over and over I'm amazed by it. I see it around me, affecting me, and yet I forget that I have the very same power on other people. What we say and do matters so much. And at the same time, we have such little power over anyone or anything. It's enough to make you crazy.

"Two people I love dearly are struggling with huge issues. The issues that are so big that the only way you get through is by locking up part of you and functioning the best way you can.

I know this one as I have done it before. It's when the world is positively crumbling and changing and if you don't hang on somehow, you will fall into the abyss. So then you hang on by turning on the autopilot mode and getting through. I know this one so well that I can sit here and actually go to that place and go to that feeling and recall what it's like clearly.

I wonder if it's ever really possible to be so okay with the losses of life that you really just accept them and don't need to close off part of yourself to get through.

I wonder if that's the goal?
I don't know.
Is it?

I gravitate toward the goal of 'becoming love.'

What the heck does that mean?

I think I need to really sit with that and get it more concrete.

Maybe the goal is 'becoming knowing.'

If you know...if you know it's all okay, that losses, change, sorrow are all part of the journey, if you know somehow it's all part of the deal...

and if you believe that there is a sacredness mixed into that deal...

Maybe then you won't close off part of you. Maybe opening all of you to all things is becoming love? Opening, embracing it all, holding the sacred, maybe somehow that's being love.

I have a quote that totally comes to mind:

'maybe it's not about the darkness.
and maybe it's not about the light.
maybe it's about the knowing.
the knowing there is sacred always.
even when you can't see it.
maybe it's the knowing that's the holy part.'

I have no idea...but I sure am curious."

So I watch. I watch people I love struggle with really big things. Sometimes I can flip their struggles on my own life stuff and learn a thing or two. Sometimes I carry the weight of their struggles way too much and have to work hard at letting go, and sometimes I know that it's all okay and will go wherever it goes.

"I spent years and years and years - and years - trying to help, pulling my hair out in frustration, thinking on it forever and crying an awful lot. I really felt I had some good answers. Still think that I did. Thing is, they're good answers for me. They work for me. No one else is me. Everyone else needs their own answers.

I think I finally figured that out with this. I mean, for real – in my bones kind of thing.

But I still don't have this detachment in other areas of struggle in my life. I still somewhere deep down think my answers are the right ones, and other people really need to just come to their senses. Yeah, I'm laughing. Yeah, well, good luck with that one, Ter.

So what's the difference here? How come I have it in one situation and not in another? I want to say that I got it kicked into me in this situation. But truth is, it should have been kicked into me in these other situations also. There was definitely kicking involved.

Maybe I need something from the situations I struggle with.

Of course I do.

Or there wouldn't be a struggle.

Maybe I don't really need anything anymore in those situations though.

Maybe I'm just in the habit of thinking I need something.

That seriously feels way more right. I'm just in the habit of thinking I need something.

And this morning, for a moment here, I can see real clearly that I don't need anything from these situations. What I do need is to have that insight sink on down into my bones."

If I can remember that it's a journey and that people are going to go where they choose to go regardless of what my thoughts are, and at the same time if I can remember that my words have incredible power, I can blend that all together to be truly helpful. I don't have to give advice, that's not helpful. I can remind people with my words that they matter. I can create safe spaces with my words for people to rest in and think in and to become more of who they are in. I can offer kindness and compassion and I can concentrate on the power that lies within that space.

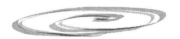

85

she suddenly saw it –
right in front of her –
she didn't have to convince anyone of
anything.
all she had to do was be.
just be.
the rest would take care of itself.

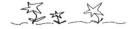

"I heard myself say it and it clicked in my mind. 'It's just a bomb waiting to go off.'

'Yeah, that was it,' I thought. Not really a new concept at all. But a visual that made total sense to me.

Thing is, there's different kinds of bombs. The inanimate ones that will go off, but there's no attachments to them. Or the human ones that carry with them so many emotional strings and entanglements that it's impossible to detach as much as you want to. But detach you must, because the closer you are, the stronger the impact.

This particular bomb has been ticking for a long time. Sometimes really quietly, sometimes so loud that I shake from the vibrations.

Here's the deal about those vibrations though. The bomb doesn't have to be ticking for me to feel them. Sometimes the bomb's mere existence has been enough to send vibrations through me.

The very threat of the explosion gets to me.
The very uncertainty of it all can make me crazy.

And I think what has happened now is that I just got real tired of shaking and waiting and losing life because of it. I think I just hit some kind of limit.

I walked and thought about it.

There's a bomb there.
Fact.

Ninety nine percent chance it will go off. Could be really bad. Could be not so bad. Could be anything. I have no control whatsoever.

All that I've been doing to try to control the impact has cost me dearly.

Time to stop. It will most likely explode. There will most likely be some definite fall out to deal with. I won't know until it happens. There are bombs everywhere in life. The blessing is that you never even know about most of them until the blow up is near you or on you.

I think of my marriage. I always say it 'exploded' because it sure felt like bombs were going off right and left. Well, I made it through. I'm happier than ever. Sometimes bombs need to shake your world to really change it. They're not all bad. They definitely aren't gentle. But they aren't all bad.

I tried to come up with good things I've gotten out of just knowing this bomb is there. Out of trying to dance around it. It took me awhile, but there were good things to see. And I saw some major growth on my part. The kind of growth I had to be pushed and pulled through, not the kind of growth I would naturally do on my own.

Okay. So I looked at this darn bomb. Fine. You be there.

And you explode when the time is right. Or when the time feels totally wrong to me. But I refuse to give up any more life to reacting to the ticking. I'm done letting the ticking drown out my own heart's singing.

And maybe that's the greatest gift that I could take away from this whole experience – that everything is a choice. And what we choose to react to is our choice. And if we choose to let something drown out our singing hearts, then we have to own that. Because that's our choice.

Do we hear the singing or the ticking?
If we hear both, which do we concentrate on?

It's entirely our choice."

recognizing her strength,
she decided to use it.

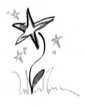

Self Doubt

She called to check in on me, she knew I had been struggling a bit. "I'm doin' way better," I told her. 'It got so bad, it kicked me into something good." And I laughed and joked about my stuff. "But YOU don't sound so good. What's up?"

There's something safe between us. And sometimes just hearing the others' voice will be enough for us to drop the shields and the tears flow right on out. I could hear her's flowing as she tried to speak. She had been on a high. She had recently finished a project that she had put her all into. It had taken tremendous commitment and effort to make it happen. And it came out beautifully. Something to feel really proud of. She had been sharing it, spreading it and rejoicing in her project. And then, something hit.

Self Doubt.

Self Doubt had landed big time and shaken her to the bone. She told me some of the thoughts that had run through her mind and what she was feeling. I sighed on my end of the phone and sank into my chair. I knew this one. Just the day before I was hearing my own voices about writing this very book. They were strong and they were loud. "What are you doing? Who are you kidding? No one wants to read this. Why are you even trying this? Put it down. Stop what you're doing. Stop being so stupid." Oh yeah, those wonderful voices that pop up.

She was crying pretty good now and her voice was shaky as she wondered why she did this to herself. She knew there was some issues buried that were surfacing, she also threw in the hormone factor, her period was due real soon, and she rounded up all the other reasons she could think of that were affecting her.

I heard the part about her cycle and grabbed that. For me, when I get my period, I get profound. There's a quiet that comes over me and I can kind of step aside and watch things a little better. I asked her if she felt similar when she had hers. She said she did. "Okay, let's say you're worn out, your hormones are funky, and there's a million reasons for this to come on now. You've got the gift of your period coming. Take it, grab it, sit with it, and listen. See if there's something you can take from this experience and use. Like maybe you can get in that profound mood and turn to those voices and tell them they're wrong. That you don't believe them. Think about what you can do now to help tweak what happens when this feeling comes to you again in the future. What can you do now as preventative maintenance for the next time this comes crashing in?"

This caught her attention. "You need to put this in your book," she said. I laughed and agreed. I don't know a person alive who isn't affected by these darn self doubt voices. And like my friend's today, they sometimes come crashing down on us so hard. "I'm okay with the ups and downs of life," she said, "I just wish the downs weren't so down." No kidding.

I suggested we be a safe place for each other. The place we go to to remind each other of our value and to pull each other back. We both have male partners and while both of them would be there for either one of us, I'm not sure they get the depths of what this feels like sometimes. I'm not sure men carry this the same as women. Maybe they do. I don't talk to enough of them to know. But I do know that having someone who really understands this, who goes through this too and who is willing to remind you over and over again of your beauty and your talents is total gold.

She's a musician. She writes and plays gorgeous music. "Can you write yourself a song?" I asked her. Can you write something to yourself that answers that self doubt?

"And sing it to myself?" she asked. Not sure of the whole deal.

"Yeah! Sing it to yourself, and let it sink inside of you."

She liked the idea and had to get off the phone quickly as lyrics had started coming to her! I smiled as I hung up and thought "I cannot wait to hear this. Every woman on the planet will need this song."

I'm not sure what the reasons are for self doubt, but I am sure it does so much damage to us. It limits us and prevents us from offering who we are. We need to work with it, tweak what we do with it, face it, tell it it's wrong, and take the power away from it, one step at a time, until it's gone and we shine in the light of the knowing our worth.

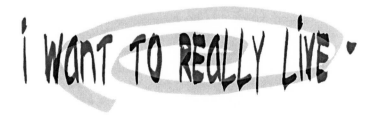

i want

i want to really really live.
i want to laugh til my stomach tightens so much
that it aches and my legs hurt
from my slapping them.
i want to cry from my gut
and let the tears wash me to where i need to go.
i want to hear the singing of my heart,
and let the sounds echo inside me
and i want to dance to that music.
i want to fill with compassion and touch
someone's face so gently that they can feel
the caring in my fingertips.
i want to love so deeply that my cells vibrate
with it and just standing near me you can
feel the buzz of the vibrations.
i want to know that i'm worthy and good
and i want to leave self doubt on the highway.
i want to touch the sky
and recognize my soul in it.
i want to walk in the rain
and drop to my knees in gratitude
for this gift of life i have been given.
may i never ever forget what a gift it truly is.

A week later I found myself hit all over again.

It kind of creeps up on me sometimes. Where I don't even really know what's going on, and then I get so knocked down flat that I can't get up. That's what's happening right now. Except I'm defying it. I'm going to write about it even as it tells me I can't. I'm not exactly 'up' yet...but I'm leaning up on my elbows, anyway.

I don't know what spurred on the first bout of self doubt, but it came through. I thought that I beat it. And yet, I didn't write again after that. I kept telling myself it's because I was busy or not quite inspired yet, or some other reason. I couldn't admit the self doubt had snagged me.

And then, a series of events over the past week have left me lost and sad. Maybe I should give up the book. Who needs it? I'm not going to do it. I don't need to do it. I'll write other things, other ways. I can't let my heart out this much. I don't want to share this much of myself. I was crazy to think I did.

I was cooking dinner. Music. I could use some music. I turned on my friend's CD. Her very first song is co-written by another friend, a mutual friend of ours. It's one of my favorites. I love that it has both of their energies mixed together. I listened and felt both of them there with me in the kitchen. The tears started coming as the lyrics just wrapped around me. I wiped the tears and thought of all the tears I had shared with friends that day.

I had called my surrogate mom first thing in the morning. Told her I didn't even know what was wrong, but I needed to talk to her. "You're going to think I'm crazy," I told her. "And this isn't even what it's about, and yet, somehow it is." I explained. And I went on to talk about the recent news of the Catholic Church's reaction to the child molesting that's going on. I cried about people looking the other way when there was so much hurt and damage happening. I talked of how that may even be more of a hurt than the actual molesting. I recognized that this was hitting my own buttons about my own experience with being molested, and that I just couldn't understand the lack of an uproar. And, I finished with the idea that the looking the other way, the not seeing, the not being there for people who have been so wronged was bringing up other issues for me. That a whole lot of past pains seemed to be surfacing through these news stories.

We talked of feeling powerless and how awful that feels. We talked of other things rolling around in my life that had stirred up a can of worms inside myself. We laughed, shared some love and then went back to our days.

Later, another friend wanted to connect on the phone. I turned her offer down. "I'm off center today, I'll just cry." She gave me space. Told me if I needed her, she'd be around.

It wasn't long before I asked for that call that she had offered, telling her I could use some help. We talked, and I cried a lot. I mentioned the news stuff getting to me and all the inner things that were whirling inside of me and how hurts from all directions were circling around me.

She talked of trust, pointing out that our trust gets knocked out of us when something bad happens and people aren't there, and when the people who hurt us are supposed to be good. How the world looks crazy and slanted and we don't know what to do. And she tied that in to other things I was feeling now in my life. I nodded through my tears as I listened to her words.

The conversation helped soothe me, but I still felt lost and I still felt that giving up the writing was the thing to do. But as I continued slicing up the veggies, I listened to my friend singing. I thought of my favorite songs of hers. They're about her struggles and her inner workings. The ones I love the most are the ones that reveal who she is inside. That matters to me. That makes the songs so valuable. And I thought of my writing. And how scary it is to put all this out on paper for anyone to read. How vulnerable it is. I thought of my conversations about power and how hard it is to trust. I thought of how skewed the world is. How much ugliness is mixed all through it. And how I want to bring beauty to it. I want to bring the glory of getting through the darkness. I want to bring the light of my heart to the world. Even though it scares the daylights out of me. I want to offer my heart.

And so, I'm here. Typing away like a fiend. Determined to stand back up and to dive back in. Because that's all I can do. That's all I can offer. Over and over again I can get up and offer myself. Because that's what I have.

I thought of the past hurts, the issues with being powerless and losing people who aren't there for you, of people not seeing, not even looking...I thought of all that pain. And then I thought about what I want. And what I want to give. Of seeing people, of really looking, and of celebrating them. Of looking at myself, really seeing me, and celebrating me. All we have is what's inside of us. If we let that pain stop us and keep us from moving forward and offering ourselves, we let that stuff win.

"Life can hurt a ton. But if we let that hurt shape our beliefs and color our outlook, we've lost ya know? I'm not much of a competitive person. And I don't really see life like a battle. But I do think we can win or lose something here. And I don't know...I just don't want to lose."

"...That led me to think about strength and power. I do believe the 'bad guys' can win. That's a fairly new belief of mine, and one that has come hard and shaken me to the core. But now, instead of wallowing in the fear of that thought, I am turning to questions that can get me somewhere with it all.

How much can they take? How much do they win? Maybe that's where the power is. And maybe that's all we ever have control over"

~~~

"It's entirely up to me what I do inside myself. No one else has the power to knock stuff outta me because I have the power to keep it in me."

~~~

"When we push ourselves to offer ourselves...to offer our light, or offer our love, or work on opening our hearts, or whatever the bottom layer is for us that we want to do...maybe that's when we push past the self doubt barriers.

And maybe just that – just pushing past the self doubt and moving into our true selves – maybe that's what we have to offer. Even though we think it's things like offering love or light or open hearts. Maybe it's just offering us.

Because...oh man...that's what we are, isn't it? Light. Love. Open hearts.

That's ultimately what we are.
Once we lose the self doubt."

the fear won't help save what you have –
it will make you lose what you could become.

I have so many fear moments it's crazy. One of my favorite fear moment stories is the story of how the bone sigh called 'living passion' was born – well, actually, it's how bone sigh arts was born! I believe they were born the same night.

I knew my marriage was ending and that it would be up to me to support myself and my sons. I had been a home-schooling/stay-at-home mom for my sons' entire lives. I wanted to keep that going. I wanted to keep their lives as stable as possible.

At the time, I was in a woman's therapy group. The women in the group were well aware of my situation and knew that I had been considering child care as a means of support. Every day I walked and thought and cried and looked up at the sky asking what I should be doing. Those moments brought me to a strong feeling. I could feel a push inside me to start an art business.

We need to take a side story here. I wasn't an artist. I hadn't always wanted to have an art business. It wasn't like I was following a dream. What had happened was I had started writing these little snippets of things to get through the painful moments of the marriage falling apart. I felt like everything was my fault, that I was ruining everyone's lives and the guilt and pain were tremendous.

What I really wanted to do was drink. It was so tempting to me. It would just take the pain away and then I'd be able to get through it all. But I had kids. I knew that I couldn't choose that way to cope. I decided that I was going to walk through this experience and not try to numb it, but try to feel it. And, oh man, at times the pain felt like just too much to hold. It would just rip my insides apart. I needed to pour it out somewhere. I turned to pouring it out in words. That's how the bone sighs were born. Whenever the pain was too intense, I wrote.

And then one night, I came home from a marriage counseling session. Those sessions were excruciating and my energy would just be completely gone by the time I got home. But this night, I wanted to make a gift for a woman in my therapy group. She was starting a new life and I wanted to make her a gift for her new home she was buying. I wrote the bone sigh 'i matter' that I included in the beginning of this book. It's about a woman who figures out that she matters. I thought that I was writing the quote about the woman in my group. But when I sat back to read it, I realized it was about me. We had many of the same issues and somehow I lost myself in the writing. Maybe I wasn't ready to write about me with that particular topic, and maybe writing about her gave me the space I needed to let some of my own issues out. I don't know, but I suspect so. I painted a watercolor candle that was also the shape of the small letter 'i' and wrote the quote out next to the watercolor. I made several of them, wanting to pick the best one to give to her.

i matter

it was when she first dared to see
her truth, that the winds howled.
after a time, it strengthened her
and she spoke her truth
and the earth shook.
and when finally,
she believed her truth –
the stars rejoiced,
the universe opened,
and even her bones sang her song:
"I Matter!"

I brought one in to my individual counselor the next day. She cried when she read it. She looked at me through tears and said "Terri, you have GOT to keep writing." I knew I did too. I nodded through my own tears.

It was after that session that I started putting watercolor to the quotes I wrote. It was my way of honoring the quotes, of honoring what was inside of me. Did I think of them as art? No. I thought of them as therapy. I thought of them as life preservers.

It was in the quiet moments of the walks that I started to get the idea of trying to sell my work. Something was happening inside of me. The writing was pouring out, creating the art with them helped calm me. Maybe it was something I could do for a living. I went to my therapy group feeling about as scared as you could get.

I needed their support. I needed to lean on them. As soon as I opened my mouth to tell them about my decision, I started crying. The whole thing was so overwhelming to me and I wanted all their arms just wrapped around me. "I need your support," I stammered out through my tears. "I need you to believe in me."

Every single one of them looked at me with looks I'll never forget. They were horrified at my plan. They loved me, they cared about me. They wanted me to be safe. Each took their turn explaining to me why I needed to go with the child care. It just wasn't a good plan to try the art business yet. They advised me to do it on the side, work my way into it, make it a hobby, don't jump in and try to make a living out of it. Do what was safe.

I honestly don't remember what my response was. I knew they were saying all of this out of love. I also knew I was scared, really scared – but I was going to start an art business. When I got in my car to go home, it was dark out and it was raining. Driving through tears and rain, I pulled up to a stop light and the bone sigh 'living passion' poured out of me.

'it is not enough to find your passion...
you must dive straight into the fire
of your fear ~
where you can grab it
and hold it
until it transforms you.'

It turns out that I really didn't 'need' their support like I thought I had. Together, my sons and I created a business that not only supported us but taught us and grew us beyond anything we could have hoped for. There are many fear stories mixed in after this one, but this is one of my favorites. I listened and followed and believed. And it worked. No one will ever be able to take that away from me. That night changed me forever. I dove straight into the fire of my fear, and I was transformed. I wonder how I knew when I wrote that bone sigh. That's the thing...those quotes aren't mine. If I'm lucky, I live my way into them.

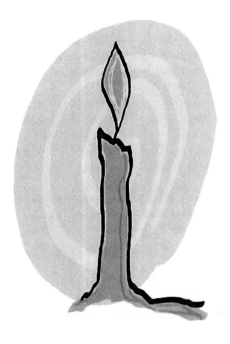

It's been quite an interesting journey starting bone sigh arts and keeping it going. In the beginning there was so much desperation and rawness to the whole thing. I'm not sure the question ever really was IF we were we going to pull it off or not, but more HOW were we going to pull it off. There was no doubt in my mind we had to make it work. And I think that had a lot to do with us actually making it. I knew nothing about business or art or much of anything. There was definitely a buzz of energy going on all the time as everything had to be learned. Throwing up my hands and asking the Universe for help was routine, putting things out there and then stepping into trust was just part of the daily deal.

And then we kind of settled into the flow and got comfortable. We were making it.

I like comfortable. I don't have a problem with comfortable. Comfort is a good thing. But maybe I don't grow as much when I'm in that zone. Okay, I know I don't. And now I'm remembering that.

Times have been tough lately and I'm watching the changes in myself. I have lost that comfort buffer, I have revisited the feelings of uneasiness and concern, and now I seem to have entered back into that starting territory I once knew so well – raw.

Raw. That's a great word and really does seem to describe how I feel.

Raw isn't necessarily bad. In fact, it doesn't seem bad at all right now. What is raw? It feels almost like there's a big sore inside of me. It's open, with tremendous potential, but it's not an easy open kind of thing, it's a touchy open. It can either become infected and turn bad or heal into something that's beautiful. It's a feeling that there needs to be careful consideration as to what will bring out the good things in this rawness. And there's tremendous determination inside to help it to its full potential. It's odd to think of it as a sore. But yeah, I think that's what it feels like.

Someone likened it to 'fire in your belly' and I smiled when I heard that. Yeah, I think there is fire in my belly again. And I think the fire comes from that sore spot.

I don't know how it works for others, but I felt that fire get lit the other day. I actually felt it. I had been in the realm of worried, concerned, bummed, trying to trust and keep moving forward. It was sort of a mid-way realm. Half way between worlds with a sort of lethargic fog hanging around.

And then I did my finances for the year. Added my numbers. And compared them with past numbers. Oh. Not good. Not good at all. And then, right then, as my index finger moved over the written numbers on the page, I felt it. The embers grew warm, and I could feel it. I turned to my computer and typed an email to my sons and my partner, and I told them what was going on. It wasn't a panicked note. It was a 'this is the scoop' note, and I felt the flame inside of me ignite. I typed 'I'm in warrior mode, and we will get through this.' And the flames burst through me.

That day I felt more alive than I had in ages. I dived into things with a renewed energy. "Two feet in," I told myself. Two feet in.

Again, I don't know how it works for anyone else, but I do see patterns happening in my own life. One of those patterns is that when I feel I get some sort of lesson or insight, it's tested almost immediately.

Sure enough, within hours, I heard the news that someone close to me was gravely ill. It threw me to the ground, scared me, worried me, weighed on me. I wobbled. I thought of my own life and how short it is even if I'm lucky enough to hit old age. What am I doing with it? What about some other things in my life? My relationships? How I'm choosing to spend my time. The doubts crept in.

I thought if I could just talk to my partner, I'd feel better, I'd understand more, I would get a grip. I'd still be scared, worried, sad, and heavy with the news...but maybe I wouldn't have that self doubt. And true to the pattern of my life, that plan totally flopped. I not only didn't get the answers I was looking for, I got more self doubt. Apparently, I wasn't going to get what I needed from an outside source. It doesn't seem to work like that for me.

I found myself wandering around my studio reading the notes I have tacked all over my walls. I could feel echoes inside of me as I read. Some of the notes made me laugh, some made me cry, one made me ache inside. All of them added to some vague echo that I couldn't quite make out.

And then it came to me. The flame inside. I felt it. It roared up again. That rawness at the base of it. The feeling of having to jump two feet in. Of there being no other choice. Of living all I can while I've got the chance. Of going full speed ahead into offering who I am.

it was time for two feet in,
a jump with both feet
and a knowing it's where she belonged.

"Living what you want in a good moment is a delicious piece of cake. Living what you want after a gut punch is empowerment."

~~~

"It's way too easy to get distracted with things that don't matter. Way too easy to let stupid things get you down.

I look out at the snow as I type and my eyes just well with tears. There's way too much beauty to hold. I can't even hold a fraction of it if my hands are empty and willing. How can I hold any of it if my hands are filled with things that don't matter?

Dustin' off my hands and holdin' them out to the Universe...fill me with beauty today. I'll hold it as best I can. I'll try, anyway."

~~~

"The concept of creating your reality has taken hold of me the last few days. The idea that everything you do matters and how you do it matters. The idea that you create the peace or turmoil around you and in you. The power that you have over your own daily existence just to make it pleasant or not. The power that you have beyond that.

I think we're both totally powerless and totally powerful. And I think that must be true as the truths seem to be the things that hold the opposites equally.

I'm aware of these thoughts/concepts, have tinkered with them before. This time though, they caught my eye and I haven't been able to put them down.

I don't want to either.

I want to keep this stuff in the front of my mind right now.

Gratitude versus entitlement came up last night. I liked that phrase. It seems to - bam - put things in their place in my mind.

Am I being grateful or am I feeling entitled?

~~~

What are we creating?

What are we putting out there?
What are we offering?

I'm thinking that little check-ins on that with myself would be a good idea.
It's almost like a weird form of praying.

What if I asked myself that every day? Like a prayer? And what if I held
those questions as sacred? And what if I viewed my answers to them as
holy? Hmmmmm..."

it is in the commitment to trust
that mountains begin to move.
it is in the commitment to love,
that walls begin to crumble,
and it is in the commitment to one's self
that worlds unimagined begin to become real.

"Offer your best.
Give your all.
Then rejoice with the ones who see it.
And bless the ones who don't.
And keep goin' forward."

~~~~~

"How is it that we let our souls get eaten away without running to save them?
Is it because it happens so slowly we don't even notice?

What are the warning signs?
Are they the same for everyone?

And when we do discover it – what then?
Do we throw security to the wind and claim our lives back?
Or do we hand it all away for health insurance and retirement funds?

I'm not accusing or mocking.
I'm seriously wondering.

Having fallen apart recently with my own health insurance crisis and then
having run straight to the most secure answer I could find, which luckily
didn't work out, I totally understand the urge to cover ourselves in security.

I'm thinking maybe it's just because we can't do the long term seeing.
We THINK we are.
We THINK we're doing the long term seeing by planning retirements and
insurance costs.

But are we seeing how quiet and subdued our souls are growing?

Is anyone noticing?"

grab your spirit. grab your heart.
hold it, hold it close, hold it up high.
let it shine
believe in it.
love it. nurture it. share it. grow it.
and never ever give it up, label it, or change it
to make someone else happy.

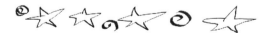

"I feel filled with defiance.
I'm not going to be who they are.
I cannot live like that.
This is it.
The gift is now.
Fill it with love.
Live that love.
Breathe that love.
Focus on what matters.
Tell the people in your life they are everything to you and back that up
with what you do.
What the heck would we wait for?
The time is now.
My God, open your eyes and see.
Open your heart and know.
If I could just scream this at the top of my lungs.
If we all could just hear it.
Why, why, why don't we hear it?
Please, God, let me hear it.
Let me live it."

~~~

"If you lose your sense of life and passion to keep from hurting – what have
you gained?"

~~~

"What matters is that we have to keep offering what's inside of us.
We have to.
Because what's inside each and every one of us is the stuff that will change
the world.
And sometimes the Universe isn't going to tell you that.
Sometimes you just have to know it.
Sometimes you just have to live it."

"At the end of every random thought, I seemed to come to the same thing. This same thought has been on my mind for weeks now.

Live it now.
Live it fully.
Be present.
Embrace the gift.

Trust has been the other theme with me that will run rampant, end thoughts and be all I can come up with as any kind of answer to anything.

I haven't combined them yet. They've been separate thoughts at separate times.

But I'm thinking – the time has come to combine them.
To filter all my thoughts with both these concepts.
Ohmygosh. Can you imagine if I could???"

Enough great insights and ideas have come to me in the shower, that I now refer to my shower as The Psychic Phone Booth. I have had so many instances of things just landing in my mind out of the blue, that I try to pay careful attention when I hear those things. A lot of times it will be an idea for something to do with my work or my personal life.

One time, though, I felt I got an entire message about how to live my life. I got out of the shower and immediately wrote it down. In recording it here, I refer to myself, but just as it is with everything in this book, the idea is to take it and turn it towards you if it seems to fit at all.

"There is stuff going on that I cannot comprehend and don't need to.
The parts I can see scare me because they threaten me in some of my most vulnerable spots.

Drop the fear.
I am loved beyond anything I can imagine.
It's a love that's beyond us, that surrounds us, that is inside all of us.

Being loved is something that exists in spades and there's no need to fear the lack of that. I do not need to see it manifested around me in particular people.

It's there.

See it or not.

I need to know that in my bones, trust it, and offer myself with a full and open heart to this stuff that's going on that I can't comprehend.

If I don't trust it, I will find myself in fear.

When I'm in fear, I won't be able to open the way I'm needed to open right now.

So trust is vital.
An open heart is vital right now.

Give it and you will not regret it.

Give it and you will give life.
Give it and you will get life."

106

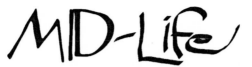

MID-Life

It had been four years since I'd seen my dad. He lived forty-five minutes up the road, and it had been four years. He was uncomfortable with my decision to divorce and he had decided it was easier not to see me. I had invited him down several times; he declined each time. He made it clear to me that he couldn't deal with me then and that he needed space. I tried so hard to give him that, even as it ripped at my insides. We traded emails one day where I told him I understood and I wouldn't push him. He seemed grateful for that. I felt like it was an odd gift I was giving him, allowing him that space with as much grace as I could. The misunderstandings floating around with family members only made something that hurt so bad seem even worse. It was a sad mess that I had hoped would work itself out.

My dad had started showing signs that something wasn't quite right with his health. The family started buzzing with concern. I was on the outside looking in now, but even I heard the questions and concern.

I met with my mom for coffee to check in. She urged me to come visit, and all I could think of was my dad telling me not to. Respecting his wishes seemed to be the only thing I could do for him. I wasn't sure what to do. I told her that I would ask him what it was that he wanted. And so I did. The holidays were coming, I asked him if we could we get together for the holidays.

True to his nature, he was honest and up front and told me that mixing the holidays and dealing with me would be too much for him. But after the holidays, I could come for a visit. A break through, I thought. It wasn't perfect, and it sure didn't feel real good to be considered something to deal with...but it would be a start.

Or not.

One morning while having tea with a friend, there was an announcement over the loud speaker. I had an emergency call. I got up, went behind the busy counter, picked up the phone and listened as my son told me that my father had a stroke. I quickly told my friend, gathered my things, and headed off to a whirlwind of saying hello and goodbye to my dad as I watched him slip away and die.

He couldn't talk at the end. In fact, there was only a brief time where I know he even recognized me and it wasn't a long look of love either. I appeared to agitate him all the way to the end. There were no lose ends tied up, there was no great ending where my father handed me his love. I spent some time alone with him handing him mine. And then he was gone.

And there I was, stepping right into what I like to call my mid life crisis. Only I didn't know it yet. The stage had been set before my dad died. Months before, I watched a heartbreaking story play out in one of my friends' lives. I had been so sure that love would win and make everything okay in her situation. But as I watched a five year old girl get court ordered back into a life of abuse in the ghetto, something shattered inside of me. My belief in good always winning blew out my veins and left me bleeding.

I was standing in that blood when my dad passed away and my mid life awakening truly began. I still didn't know it. It took a long time of searching and feeling crazed inside before I picked up a book that gave me that 'aha' moment. Ohmygosh. I'm in a mid-life passage. The relief was huge. I suddenly remembered that the darkness would bring gold. I had forgotten that darkness does that. I remembered that it was a journey, and that I was finding more and more things I needed to find. And to find those things, I needed to let go of what no longer worked for me. Including many of my beliefs.

"Maybe, I thought, maybe mid-life is when you've seen too much, and your control freak can't control anymore. You can only fake the control beliefs for so long before they start falling apart. Maybe mid-life is when your inner control freak gets crippled.

And maybe the struggle I feel through this time of life in trying to find my beliefs and purpose is directly related to the thrashing about that my inner control freak is doing.

I thought of my friends and my family. I don't control them. But I can get overwhelmed with wanting to fix everything for them. Yeah, that would be control. The idea of suffering and dying – shoot, I'm just not good with that. Again, control stuff. It runs rampant through me. But not in the obvious ways. And that inner control freak is really feeling crippled.

I'm thinking my beliefs are based in this stuff. Wow, what a weird feeling to even really consider that my actions, my beliefs, my emotions that I allow in, are all based on my system of control.

And I control that system. And what's controlling the controller?
Oh my goodness, have I got some thinking through to do.

Feel every feeling.
Don't filter.
Don't control.
Giving it a try..."

it's not about controlling
it's about being present,
being open
being aware –
and allowing it to come.

"And I landed right smack in the middle of the 'what's it all about?' place.

What the heck IS it all about???
What's the point?
Why are we here?
Does it matter what we do?

The only thing that makes any sense to me is the candle theory.

The candle theory is the idea that there's one main flame somewhere and that we've all got candles inside us lit from that main flame. Our job is to grow that flame. To make it shine brighter.

That's still my theory of choice. Even though the 'main flame' part has changed forms in my mind, taking on more of an energy feel over the years, it's still my theory of choice.

But so what? I asked myself that this morning. So what? So you die and your flame's bright(er). So?

And then I asked myself some other questions. Does it matter who we love? Does anything last? Is anything worth giving your all for? And I felt like I knew the answers to these questions, although, I don't know why.

It does matter who we love. While we have to love all that we can as much as we can, (I think) the ones you really give your heart to matter.
That affects everything. That affects growing your flame.
Love lasts. It's the only thing I know that does last.
It IS the flame.
And love seems to be the thing worth giving your all to.
Why?
I don't know.
It's just a feeling I carry around inside."

109

she couldn't control events.
only her heart.
and it was to her heart
she wanted to give freedom.

"Sooner or later we're all going to get the rug pulled out from under us. Maybe some of us will have it pulled out fast enough we won't even know, but a lot of us are going to be sitting there rugless, waiting to die.

WHY would we build a lifetime of stuff that doesn't matter? WHY would we create a world that won't support us in the darkness? Question after question was whirling inside of me last night.

And when you look at it that way, it's not courage that makes you want to build 'real' is it? It's just kind of like planning ahead or something. It's like building the foundation that will last.

It's not about courage.

And all that fear that I encounter along the way in trying to be real? That fear is just roadblocks or something. Whenever you REALLY look at stuff you're afraid of, it's really not that scary. I think it's scarier not to look and then have it all land on you at the end.

THAT'S scary!

So maybe somehow we've got it all backwards? And maybe if we could just turn it all around, it wouldn't be so hard.

Yeah, right.

It's the turning it all around stuff that takes some work, huh?

I don't know...but I do know this...I'm not on this journey of searching because I'm courageous. That I know.

I'm on it because I want real. And not having real is way scary for me.

So, I guess I'm on this journey because I'm chicken!"

it was when she casually mentioned
"fake happiness" that my world stood still.
i knew what she meant all too well.
i had lived it.
become it.
it was time for Real.
i want real happiness.
need it.
deserve it.
demand it...
take it!

"Something's hit me that I haven't figure out yet. Which means I shouldn't write about it yet, but would a confused mind ever be enough to stop my ramblings?

It's the mid-life thing. The changes that happen. And no, I don't mean the physical changes. The inside changes. It's the seeing things differently. More clearly for what they are. Sometimes that's really cool. And sometimes it's enough to make my bones tremble.

I think maybe part of mid-life is really leaving the childhood visions of things behind. Please understand me, I don't mean leave the child-like wonder and excitement behind. I never want to leave that behind. But the child-like easy answers, the child-like perceptions of people, those things need to be left behind.

Because answers aren't always easy. And sometimes they just aren't what we want to see. I think part of the mid-life passage, and I'm guessing as I'm only on one side of it so far, is that I will see things for what they are. And my bones will tremble.

And maybe I'll know I passed through and made it to the other side when my bones stop trembling and when I can just do that wise nod and say 'Yep. That's the way it is.' and not tremble.

But I'm thinking I can't get there without first seeing the stuff I don't want to see. I've been covering my eyes because I can't believe it. I have to peek through my fingers and look again. I have to pull my hands from my face and really see. Even if seeing makes me tremble.

I'm in the peeking through my fingers stage and doing a little trembling. Before I would have said I had to hold it all a bit. But now I know I'm going to have to get a clear vision and really know what I'm seeing and then I'm going to have to let it pass through me. Let it run right through my insides, touching my heart as it passes and then letting it run back out to the world.

I've got a plan now. One that may very well get me to that wise nodding one of these days. I've got some seeing to do. Some trembling to do. Some flowing to do. And eventually, some accepting to do. Life is never dull."

like the rings of a tree
marking it's growth,
the ripples of honesty that
circled thru her life
marked hers.

"An author I'm reading mentioned that when you give up a belief that's been part of you, the normal reaction to the giving up is sadness.

It can get out of hand and all that...but sadness and depression, that's okay. It's normal.

I was working and feeling the sadness and just letting it flow through me. It wasn't until I hit the shower that I remembered what I had read.

And yeah, I am giving up a belief. And he says that is important. That we have to do that constantly throughout life in order to grow. We have to give up little pieces of ourselves and change and grow. It's part of the deal.

And yeah, I'm growing, and yeah, I lost a belief recently, and yeah, it's made me really, really sad. But that's normal!

It's a process.
It's a growing.
It's a changing.

there is no map
you gotta write your own.
you gotta carve your own.
you gotta sweat, cry, grieve,
laugh, and love your own.
and when you've all done,
that's all that will have mattered.

I try to remember to get into the flow. The flow. That darn stinkin' flow. When I feel like I'm in it, I'm happy, strong, powerful, feelin' groovy. When I wrestle with being out of it, trying to get back in, or ignoring the fact that I believe there even IS a flow, well, I don't do so good. For me, the hardest part is whether I'm in that flow or not is totally up to me. I don't like to believe that. I'd much rather sit screaming on the side of the road "HOW DO I GET BACK IN?!!" and hope someone stops and takes me there. But deep down, I know it's my deal.

"How does one step into that next stage of life with consciousness, with purpose, with intent...without totally freaking out and digging in her heels and screaming 'I'M NOT GOING!!!??!'"

~~~~~~~~

"There is no one answer. It will change daily or by the moment. I just need to follow my heart as I go along. There's no one answer that will fix this for me. Trust my heart."

~~~~~~~~

"It's not a 'just do this and it'll be fine' kinda life, is it? It's a constant embracing, letting go, embracing, growing, changing, let it go, change it again kinda thing. One thing leads to another."

~~~~~~~~

"Sometimes I don't know how to hold it all, I thought. So don't, I answered as I hopped over the ditch in my yard. Don't. Just open to it. And let it flow through you. Turning, I looked back at the gray, wet morning. Let if flow through you, Ter. Let it flow right on through."

"I've heard the 'you can't go back, you can't stop time, the world can't stand still' stuff forever. But I really saw it this morning. It's hard to let go of things that were wonderful at some point. But it's the very definition of life, isn't it? It's not about holding on to. It's about flowing with. It is in the holding that I stop living. Just as it is in the flowing that I truly am alive."

~~~~~~~~

As I sat on my front porch having a cup of tea and watching the sky, I had a thought. Something had happened the night before. Without knowing it at the time, I realized I had stepped back into some power of mine. I claimed something that was deep inside of me. And I claimed it out loud. For me, there's something vital about the 'out loud' part. As I sat there drinking my tea, I realized that I felt empowered. And I realized I hadn't felt empowered in a long time.

"I watched the birds land in a tree across the street, and I wondered. Do I need to feel empowered to touch the flow? Maybe I just need to feel strong in myself? Not exactly empowered, but good about myself, confident - that kind of thing.

I argued with myself over this one. The time in my life when I felt the most like I was in tune with something beyond me, when I felt a trust in life's process and a knowing that I was going in the right direction, when I felt in the flow, was during one of the hardest times of my life. Guilt and shame and a whole host of really un-empowering feelings filled me. And yet, I lived inside a flow that was beyond me. How does that fit in?

I did feel guilt and I did feel shame, and at the same time, I was doing what I had to for me. I was taking care of me. I knew my life was unhealthy and I knew I had to go in another direction. Even if that was excruciating to go through and even if I wobbled all the way along, the very act of taking my life back was about as powerful as I could get.

So, yeah...I was empowered. I just didn't know it. And yet, it was at that time I wrote the following bone sigh:

she took her power back – without permission."

On some level, I knew it. And I'm thinking that it does matter. That when the inner strength is up on the upper levels, up top, when there's some sense of knowing you're going in the right direction, when you stop and hear your heart and then ACT on it, then you step into the flow.

That's so basic. How come that goes by me all the time?!

When you stop and hear your heart and act on it, when you live your days doing that, there is a flow.

"I don't know what any of it's about. But equally as strong as this confusion of mine, is my belief in an energy called 'Love' that is beyond anything I can comprehend. I don't see any other answer but to throw up my hands, crinkle my face in confusion, take a deep breath, and step into love.

Here's the kicker though...

If that's what I think it's all about, and if that's what I think is at the bottom of it all somewhere, somehow, then I can't just mindlessly say 'yeah, yeah, I'm in.' If I do that, I'll miss the journey. The real journey. 'Cause that's just lip service.

I may not know what it is. And I may not know what it's about. But I do know it's two feet in or forget it.

Two feet into something you don't understand and something you don't know where it goes to... and yet, you're supposed to jump with two feet in??

Yeah. I think you are. I believe people refer to that as the 'mystery' of it all."

Two feet in and following your heart. That is where I started out years and years ago when I first turned to take my power back. And I think somehow the chaos and the uncertainty of it all actually was a catalyst into the trust. You either hung on for the ride, or fell into oblivion. And I had no choice then, I had kids counting on me. I had to hang on for the ride.

And then, I think it's interesting what happened. I started getting more comfortable, things settled down a bit, I could see we were going to get through the darkness. I was settling in. And then bam! And bam again! And then bam yet again! I got hit over and over with some pretty big punches.

What I'm curious about is the timing. If I wasn't comfortable, if I was still in the chaos mode, would I have ridden the tidal waves any better? Would I have been coming at them with the strength of living 'in the flow' that I had been living in? Or did the comfort I slip into also slip me out of the flow somehow and make me even more unprepared for the flood? I have no idea. It seems like a crazy idea to think chaos would have made coping with more chaos easier. But I do wonder. I just know there was an undertow, there were tsunami waves, there was pulling from the depths, there was water crashing everywhere, and I went under.

"There are some beliefs about life that I picked up really young that are just really wrong. But I didn't know. And now they're seeped into my bones. Trying to get them out is tough. Things like, 'People come into your life and stay.' Or "Life is constant and steady.' Or the idea that if you work at things to make them good, create the white picket fence kind of thing, you'll be all set, there will be a happily ever after. That stuff.

Oh. And don't forget this big one, 'Good always wins.'

If you've got those things in your bones, it can mess with your system. At least it does with mine.

And maybe getting those wrong beliefs out is the wrong focus. Maybe getting the beliefs in is what I need to focus on. Because if they settle into my bones, the wrong ones will just have to move on over. And out.

Life IS change.
Life IS flow.
There is nothing stagnant about it.
People come in for a time, and then they go.
There is no happily ever after. But there are some deeply happy times on the journey filled with all kinds of emotions. The good things you share with people never die. People do. But love doesn't. And THAT'S what you can hold on to. Good doesn't always win. But good CAN move mountains. Love CAN change things. And good touches in ways you can't know. And through it all, the only way to survive is to be able to release your grasp. Release your grasp, and flow."

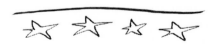

trust walked up to opening
and gently tapped her on the shoulder.
may i have this dance? he asked.
smiling shyly, she wrapped her arms
around him.
whirling to the rhythms,
melding with the music,
they dance their way into truly living.

"I think I trip myself up all the time wanting to have one answer to every situation. It doesn't work that way, does it? There's not one answer. There's a bunch of different answers that change with the moments. They're fluid. They're misty. They're downright foggy sometimes. As I walked and thought of this, I saw the mist clearing and the blue sky coming out. I smiled. To be open to it all...that is what I think I might need to be doing. Opening to it all."

it was her heart she needed to open –
not the door.
the door was wide open –
all she needed to do was dare.

"Something has been dawning on me lately. I've been sitting with it a bit. The more I sit with it, the more it feels right. I call it 'The Yin Yang Principle.' It's when you've got the opposites going and both are true. Well, it's finally sinking into my bones that life isn't a Disney movie. I know, I'm slow. And what you have is a huge mix of the joyful and the sorrowful, and you can have both at the same time. I think I have used up so much energy just fighting the 'sad' or the 'bad' and trying for it all to be good. But there's no reason for the fight.

It's never all one thing. It's always a mix. So the practical application for me goes something like this: I work on holding both. While holding both, I concentrate on the one that fits the moment. There's a time for both. To hold just one is wrong. It's not whole. I hold both, but at different moments, and know that at every given moment, there is both.

I've tried it out just a bit so far, and I'm amazed at how much it's helping me. I'm thinking the more I practice, the more I'll be able to go from one to the other. I'm thinking I'm on to something here. And I'm really liking it.

Life. That ol' yin yangy thing."

totally new territory
with not even a piece of a map,
surrounded by fear too big to hold,
a whisper begins to echo thru my mind,
thru my heart.
'release.'
'surrender to the moment.'
'be'

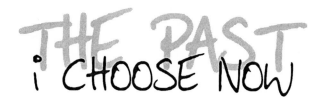

i CHOOSE NOW

the past rose up with incredible strength
pulling me away.
opening my eyes,
i focused on your face
and whispered thru tears
'i choose you.'
and the past faded away.

Recently, through several different conversations with friends, I realized I had come quite a distance in my acceptance of things in my past. I had been working on walking through the pain and trying to understand what was going on and how it all worked for years. Years and years and years. But it wasn't until I heard myself with my friends that I realized I had made major progress. I took a walk and thought about it. I wasn't just 'okay' with what had happened and the scars that I carried, I was grateful those scars were there.

Grateful? How totally odd is that? But I am. I truly understand, for the first time beyond my head and into my bones, that those scars and memories are part of who I am now. And I like who I am now. And I wouldn't trade those lessons I learned for anything.

Those scars have added to my depths. My compassion is deeper, my strength is deeper, my passion for what I do is deeper, my entire life is deeper because of those scars. And for that I'm grateful.

There is still much work to be done, however. Because while the past may rest quieter inside me now, it still sparks fears in the present. And those sparks need to be watched and worked with.

A conversation I had recently centered around the differences between our reactions to someone expecting us to play a role they've decided on for us, and the reactions to someone taking us for granted.

We agreed that taking someone for granted was the easier of the two. It's not a good thing, but if you care enough for each other that a gentle 'Hey, what the heck are you doing here?' is enough to get you back on track then it's not so bad. While not a pleasant thing, it is certainly workable and the trust you have in each other would keep that stuff in check.

The role playing is a horse of a different color. If I even get a whiff of a possibility of maybe a chance of someone even thinking they want me to play a role for them, I cringe, stiffen up, try to squeak out a protest, then basically go run, hide and or leave.

Why the big reaction? Why not a simple "Hey, what the heck are you doing here?' like I can do with the taking for granted problem. For me, it's my past creeping in. And if it was as simple as reacting to a warning sign then I'd say it was a healthy response. I would say it's a good thing. But it's not.

Significant people in my past loved me because I filled a role for them. I was the good whatever it was they needed. I see this all around me with people everywhere. We are the good daughters, the good wives, the good friends, the good workers, the good women. Who we are is not the issue. What we can do for these people is. Play the role, you are rewarded with their love. Step out of the role, the love takes on a whole new look.

Sounds simple enough, yet I think the ins and outs of this concept are so intricate and complicated that a lot of times we don't even know it's going on for years and years. We know we feel lonely, unseen, unfulfilled...kind of. Maybe. But maybe it's just us. Maybe we aren't doing something right. Maybe if we just fix ourselves a little bit, it will all be okay.

It took me a lifetime to see this stuff. I saw it, broke from it, have left it behind. Or have I? Did I run so hard and so fast that I never quite really stopped running? I'm a checker now in my relationship. Check twice, three times, and check again...does he really love me or is he using me to fill some kind of need and does he even know who I am?

Well, okay, that might be fine when you first get together with someone. Be cautious, think it through. But when the person has proven themselves over and over again, maybe it's time to put the checkers on the shelf.

And my checkers don't stay on the shelf. I am lucky enough to have a person in my life who knows this, understands this, and is willing to give me some time to work through this. But I need to grab it and deal with it. Because that's the way your past can come creeping in and ruin your present.

122

I got a note from a friend recently describing how much her husband loved her. In their spiritual views, they had some radical differences, and he not only accepted that, he loved her for it. He loved the 'adventure' of living with her and all the new things she brought to their relationship. He saw her beauty and treasured it. I read that note and tears came to my eyes. How precious that is. While I sat there and thought about what she had said, I thought how much that matters to me. How much I want that in my own relationship. And then I smiled at myself. Do I give that to my partner? Do I let him know that his differences from me make him valuable to me? Or do I tell him that his differences scare the daylights out of me and feed my checker syndrome? Ahhhh...I have come a long way with my past, and I have a long, long way to go yet.

One day, when talking to my friends, I hope to hear myself say that I've learned to put the past completely on the shelf. To value the scars inside me, and to have left the baggage behind. I want to hear myself say that, and I want to feel that in my bones.

"And I started talking about the space he makes for me. Always. Space to wobble. Space to question and wonder. Space to learn. And if I wander too far, he calls me back. Sometimes gently, sometimes not so gently.

I'm kind of thinking space making is THE most important thing we can do for someone. I've talked about it before, it intrigues me. I've done it for people, but haven't thought much of it. Until I realized what it meant to me. It matters. A ton. It allows my growth.

What more can you do for someone than to allow their growth?

And what are you saying when you do that?

I love you.
I love who you are.
I believe in you.
I believe in your capacity to grow.
You matter enough for me not to control you.
You matter enough for me to just watch and know that you are perfect as you are.

And maybe, it teaches both people about the wonder of life...
the wonders of love."

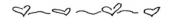

he accepted her for all she was.
always making room for her to be.
it was in that room she saw
it wasn't anyone else that needed
to accept her.
it was up to her to do it for herself.

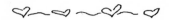

There's always those who won't see you. Always. There's always those who want you to fill a role for them. Do you want to fill your life with that? It's something we need to ask ourselves. The more I fill my life with people who really can see me and who really do love me, the easier it is for me to let go of those who cannot. I'm finding that I don't need things from them anymore.

"So there was this funky little blip in my life today. My girlfriend called, and I told her about the funky blip. She was indignant for me as she knows the whole story, and she asked "WHERE do people get the audacity they do?!"

I laughed. I told her I had been thinking about it. It had gotten quiet here. I was alone working, so I could think a bit. And I don't think it took 'nerve' for this person to do what they did. I think they have no capacity to see me, so they thought nothing of it. I honestly believe that.

And I don't know why, but that feels real good to be able to see that. I'm calm about it. I guess I don't need them to see. It's so cool. And I see it as a chance to be peaceful towards them. I see it as a chance to need nothing back.

It feels awesome."

watching them,
she saw their hearts and loved them.
knowing herself,
she stepped back and let them go.

"How do you stay open from a gut punch, she asked?

I don't know, I answered.
I just don't know.

Maybe you realize the gut punch wasn't about you. Sure, it LOOKED like it was about you. It SOUNDED like it was about you. It HURT like it was about you.

But maybe what you have to know is that it isn't about you. It really isn't.

Gut punches come from insecurities, weaknesses, fears, that kind of thing.

Staying open is KNOWING that.

Staying open is believing in yourself.
Knowing who you are.
KNOWING your worth.

And turning to those who also know it, and opening to them.

And to the one who threw the punch? See their insecurities, weaknesses, and fears. ALLOW them to be, and move away from them. For now, anyway.

It's the allowing them to be that's being open to them.
It's the moving away that's being open to you.
It's the healthy stuff that allows you to open your heart.

Maybe?
But then again...I just don't know."

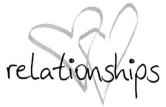

relationships

Here's a piece of gold that just landed in my life. I honestly feel this is one of the most helpful, brilliant things I've ever heard, and no, it did not come from me. The credit goes to the man in my life. This is his thought that I offer you.

I was struggling with my perception of his love for me. I wasn't feeling what I thought was love. We talked about it, and as he began to tell me what he was seeing, I felt myself relax. I could tell that he was seeing me and understanding me. In that atmosphere, I felt safe enough to ask him if he thought that I was trying to create a 'Disney movie' image of our love. To his tremendous credit, he very gently said 'yes.' And to my tremendous credit, I not only heard what he was saying, I knew it was brilliant.

He gently pointed out to me that we all carry images around for different things. In this instance, it's my image of what love should be. We carry these images around and create them for many different reasons. I know that my past hurts influence the image of love that I've created, and are also part of the reason why I hang on to that image. There is some sense of security in holding on tight to these things.

The idea, though, is that there are many different components to what it is we want. For love, my components would include things like trust, honesty, respect, acceptance, those kind of things. The components themselves are valid. But what we do with them can become a problem. Taking them and using them as pieces to a puzzle that creates one image of what we're looking for can wreak havoc in our lives. Because now we've got one picture of what love must look like, or what a good kid must look like, or what a best friend must look like, or whatever it is we've got a picture of. We've kind of lost sight of the components and just now see the one picture.

The thing is, the picture is created by us. It's no one else's picture. No one else is going to fit into it exactly. Life doesn't work that way. And the danger is that when we actually do get what we want with the components that we want but in a different picture, we will miss it, disregard it, pass it by.

Use caution with this idea though as you don't want to just accept something that looks different than that image of yours. This idea comes with the assumption that you will look deeply at what components are truly there.

127

The key is those components you started out with. Are they there in whatever is going on? And if so, are you missing them because they're being presented in a different form? And if not, are you fooling yourself into believing they are there?

I'm wondering if we can turn this idea onto everything in our lives, including our own selves. If I'm struggling with something about myself, if I'm not being who I think I want to be, have I got an image inside me that is keeping me from seeing my own beauty? That seems so possible to me. Something to definitely think about.

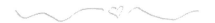

My relationship with the guy in my life definitely has its challenges. We have been a couple for years now but have put off living together for awhile yet. We both have kids to raise, and for various reasons agreed to wait on our shared living arrangements. It's a choice we have made and while we agree it's what we want, we also know that this arrangement causes certain problems. It also brings with it certain bonuses. I have had more than one friend look at my set up of two houses and living separately with envy, which makes me laugh. Relationships however, no matter what the set up, are full of challenges.

I think because of the set up, we've chosen to work really hard at what we have together. Well, because of the set up, and because we both don't want to mess up again. Having each gone through a divorce, we realize what a mess we can make of a relationship and now work really hard at keeping things on track.

After years and years of work at this, I still have a million unanswered questions about love and relationships, but I do feel like we're learning a lot as we go along. Recently, I feel like we stumbled on a golden root and landed splat into something really valuable. I wanted to try to share it. Sometimes I think it's only valuable because of our weird set up, but then I remember married life. I was married for a million years and I haven't forgotten my reactions in that situation either, and so I know this can carry over to any relationship.

I have to honestly say I don't trust my guy one hundred percent. I put that out there as I'm not sure I'll ever trust anyone one hundred percent. I might. I like to think I would. But I don't know, I think that all has to do with how much I trust myself. Seems to be all tied together somehow. But I do know there are certain areas in which I trust him one hundred percent. And one of those areas is in my belief in his good will towards me. I honestly believe that he will not try to purposely hurt me. That yes, he still hurts me, but that it's never intentional. I am pleased to say that he feels the same trust in return.

Okay, I think that's a pretty big deal. And maybe I need to stop there before I go any further. We have been through enough 'bad' times where I know it would have been easy for him, even natural, maybe, to do some slamming with his words. And yet he never has. I've seen great control in him in his responses at times, and he has never tried to hurt me. This is a big deal, because I don't think this is true of a lot of people. I've experienced enough rough times with other people trying to jab when they're threatened, that I know that not everyone exercises this control - men and women alike.

If that's something you don't have, or you, yourself, don't offer, it seems like a great thing to stop and think about and maybe work on. And if it is something you do have, do you make the most of that? I didn't. And that's what I want to share here.

I didn't do anything with that trust. Well, no, that's not true. I shared things with him that I didn't with other people. But I didn't do anything with that trust when I was feeling threatened. When threatened, I will leap into one of my defense mechanisms or modes of protection. Curling up in ball, running in the other direction, putting the walls up or shutting down, you name it, I have a nice collection of things I can do. But why would I? If I believe he didn't mean the hurt intentionally, why would I react in these ways? Why wouldn't I go to him and tell him I'm hurt, that I know I'm misunderstanding something about it, and that I'd like his help with it? Isn't that the reaction of trust? Isn't that the reaction of love?

Well, it wasn't my reaction! And recently, after weathering a rough experience together, I came to this spot where I really see that if I do trust like I say I do, then I certainly am not backing that up with my actions. And so we talked about it. And both agreed that's the goal. To believe in the other person that deeply. To know that we're safe there and that hurt is caused by misunderstandings and to work on figuring those out together.

After coming to this spot, I called a good friend, a woman friend, another person I trust to not hurt me deliberately and I told her of this conversation. I heard my voice on the phone with her, I was in awe. "Can you imagine believing in your partner this much?" I asked her. She was equally in awe and answered with a sad 'No.' I realized how lucky I was to even get to a place where I could try this with someone. I think it's huge, and if it doesn't seem huge as you're reading this, I probably have explained it badly. Because I can't think of too many places I see anyone practicing this. And I would think that we all want this in our lives. I thought it was definitely something to think about and share!

if she really believed it -
if she really trusted it -
well, then, it was time
she really lived it.

Oh, the topic of love! I have so many thoughts, blog bits, and bone sighs to share about many different kinds of love! This totally delights me because it wasn't all that long ago that I wasn't so sure that love even existed.

I knew that I had deep love for my kids, and I knew that I was capable of deep love, but as far as any more than that goes, I just wasn't sure. I can still remember exactly where I was when I figured out that what I had in my life wasn't love. I remember stopping right in my tracks in the middle of the street when the thought hit me.

People said they loved me. And what can you say to that? I guess if I'm in a generous mood, I would say that they love me in their own way. But I don't really believe that. I just say things like that sometimes to kind of ease on by the really hard stuff and keep on going. What I really believe is that the word love is used incorrectly more than it is used correctly, and that people need to examine their feelings before they go spreading the love word around. Do you even know the person that you claim to love? Do you know their thoughts and feelings? Do you see them for who they are and value that person? Or do you value who it is you want them to be? Those are some really big questions.

> they sat around me encircling me
> with compassion and wisdom.
> bandaging the wounds made in the name of love.
> over and over they claim "it's nothing."
> well, then...give me "nothing" over "love" any day.

So I started at the very beginning of it all, which was figuring out what love was in the first place. I asked everyone I interacted with, "What is love?" I was consumed with this question. It led to many interesting conversations but no answers. I could only find bits and pieces of what love must be made of. I was amazed at how little thought we've all given this question!

As I searched, something quietly was going on around me. I was surrounding myself with the very thing I was searching for. I didn't even know it, and was still denying love existed, when a shop owner I worked with asked me if I would put together some bone sighs about love for Valentine's Day. I laughed when she asked. "You're kidding, right? Me? I don't think I have any, but I'll see what I can do," I told her.

And there is another moment that will live in my memory forever. Sitting on the floor, surrounded by my writings, my bone sighs, and finding piece after piece about love. No, they weren't your typical romantic love pieces, they were pieces I had written about friends being there for me. Mostly girlfriends, a few guy friends. There was one that I wrote for a cousin getting married, so yeah, that was romantic love, and I knew that was in there. But this other stuff? I had no idea. Love had surrounded me the whole time I denied it even existed. Somehow that seems profound, kind of like a definition of love right there in that very statement.

As I gathered up the quotes, I cried. I had no idea what was in store for me in any kind of romantic way. But as far as filling my life with real love, I had done so. I had cleared out many unhealthy things, and somehow that opened a door for the healthy stuff to come tumbling on in. And tumble in it did. As it surrounded me that day in my writing, I felt my heart open like it hadn't in a long time.

i took my heart back and made it mine.
it hurt at first...
and then it sang.

Some time before my marriage split up I was consumed with the idea of passion, purity of heart and touching something beyond me. It was another time in my life where I stopped people everywhere to ask them my questions. I would ask people over and over if they knew what their passion was. And I searched inside to see if I could find what my own answers could be. My life had to explode. It had to. Looking back, I know that now. I needed to start over. I needed to clean out the stuff that wasn't real, the stuff that wasn't love, the stuff that was keeping me from touching what I really wanted to touch.

After my search for valentine bone sighs that day, I could see that I had love in my life. And I clearly had love inside of me. But there was more that I wanted. And I knew that. I wanted to touch something beyond me. I wanted to BE love.

Somehow I knew that all along.

I started talking about it here and there.

> "A buddy of mine wrote me a note after reading one of my blogs and asked me what exactly I meant by 'being love.'
>
> Oh, man. What a great question! It means I have to really think about it to even begin to try to explain it.
>
> Okay, how to even start?

131

I equate God and Love. I think there's this thing called love that we don't understand. I don't mean the romantic stuff. That can have parts of what I mean in it, but it's also so mixed with other stuff and complicated that it's not what I'm talking about.

I mean pure love.

Pure love, to me, must also somehow be God. And I really don't even know what I mean by that. I just have this feeling that all that whirls together. And I think pure love is something that we don't understand because we don't experience it very often. But when we do experience it, we know it.

I figure that it's at the core of all of us. That we all have this 'God Stuff' inside of us. And when we reach it, touch it, and live in it, that's what I would call 'being love.' The more I go along, the more I believe that being love has GOT to start in a really strong foundation of self love.

That ol' bit about you can't love anyone else until you love yourself? Well, there sure is a ton to that. And I don't think you can really touch love until you make strides in the self love department.

So, I think being love starts with self love. And then, if you can get yourself to a place where you aren't working from within a whirlwind of baggage (and I think that can only really disappear through self love) then you can operate from a really free space.

Now, see...this is all theory for me. I don't have it down! So I'm just kind of rolling with some of the things I'm learning along the way.

When I say I want to be love, I mean that I want to be able to give freely, to care and to have compassion without having the need to control or to fix, to allow things to flow and to know that everyone operates from their own place and that I can't understand it so I can't judge it. To know that it's all part of a big picture and that the little things have absolutely no meaning, and absolutely a ton of meaning all at the same time.

Being love would mean operating with an open heart and not needing to close down for protection because it would all be okay. That opening would be like a pipeline to the Universe where something beyond us flows through. It would be about keeping that pipeline clear.

Yeah...I'm no way near it.

Today I'm thinking it has to include compassion for all.

True compassion that is real and not something I know I should have, so I try real hard and come up with some sort of something that isn't quite it. But this would be something that just flows out naturally. With no need for anything back.

It would include seeing the pain of others and holding it gently and setting it down, knowing it's okay.

I would know joy in my bones. Being love has got to include joy. To be able to experience intense joy along with intense sorrow and allow both to exist side by side.

All of that is part of it.
Yeah...not so easy, huh?!

But just suppose, just pretend for a minute that was really the goal. The mission. The dream.

All my problems would look different, wouldn't they? These people I'm struggling with today, all the issues, all the challenges - all that would be different inside of me.

And if I could get there, which I don't think I can even if I had 27 life times to try...but I still want to try anyway...if I got there? Well, then, when it came time to die – wouldn't I just slip into the vastness of love that is beyond us? Wouldn't that just be awesome?

That's kind of what I like to think about sometimes. And sometimes I like to try to work on it. "

slowly, she was beginning to see it,
it wasn't about acting or thinking
or getting or giving love.
it was about breathing love,
living love –
becoming love.

"I'm not a cutter.
Never have been.
I've never even know any cutters (that I was aware of anyway) until the last seven years. Now I know about cutting in very personal ways and realize how wide spread it is. This floors me, fills me with sadness, sickness and sorrow.

That's one reason that the website 'to write love on her arms' got to me so deeply. They took the story of a young woman carving something horrible into her arm, and turned it around. They turned it around and wrote love on her arms. They are truly daring to make love their mission.

I was just writing a friend about it. How that's what we need to do. We need to write love on each others' arms. All over the place. This morning I can so easily see an arm cut and bleeding. The world's arm. And I can so easily visualize reaching out and holding it. Gently washing it, cleaning it, caring for it. Wrapping it to stop the bleeding. And gently, ever so gently taking my fingertips and lovingly outlining LOVE across the arm.

It's the world's arm. It's your arm. My arm. Her arm. His arm. I can just so feel it this morning.

It's what we need to be doing, you know?

I turn to my day and wonder how one does that with their day.

I'll listen closer.
I'll take a little longer to respond,
and I'll know how to respond because love is part of me.
All I have to do is listen.

And ever so gently, write love with my being..."

*understanding now that kindness was
the way to open her heart,
she dropped to her knees
and opened herself
to its presence.*

"I'm not sure if anyone, including my partner, really takes me seriously when I say that I'm just now learning how to love. I hear responses about my being a loving person which is really nice to hear and the intentions are good, but I feel like I'm not really getting my point across.

Yeah, I can be kind and loving towards people, but REALLY learning how to love someone is a whole different ball game.

It wasn't until I hit my forties that I even figured out that I didn't know a thing about love. It took that long to get to the point where I could see my blindness! But I am starting to learn. My eyes are open.

Figuring out that self love is totally entangled in loving others came quickly. But how open are my eyes to self love?

Thing is, self love, loving others, love stuff...none of it is 'just follow these five easy steps and before you know it – ta da! - you'll be a master of love!' There are so many subtleties to it. So many twists. And many of them go right by me. I don't even notice that I put myself aside and show way less than love to myself. How many times do I give myself away and hurt myself in the process?

Go deeper, Ter.

How many times do I believe I HAVE to do that to keep someone's love?

Go deeper, Ter.

How many times do I believe that I can't really be me because I'm not lovable?

Do I know I'm worth loving?

Right there.

Stop right there.

Is it others not loving me?
Or me not loving me?

135

Start with yourself.
You can't get anywhere until you start with yourself.

I've done subtle things to try to show myself my belief in my worthiness of love. Time to step up beyond the quiet little namby pamby actions. They're not good enough anymore. Time to say it a little louder to myself.

Time to shout it out.

Oh my. Shout?

Tell me...could you shout it to yourself?
If not – why?

Okay, maybe I'm not ready to shout.
But I am ready to get beyond a whisper. I'm ready to speak.

One step at a time."

I wonder why it's so hard for so many of us to get the self love deal down. Just yesterday I was talking to a friend on the phone, someone had given her a message that profoundly moved her. Part of the message was that she was a wonderful person, a good person, a good mom. Her voice was choked up as she was telling me about it.

It reminded me of having tea with her years before when she was telling me about some problems she was having. As we talked, we tried to dig further and further into what was really going on inside of her. And there, across the table from me, the tears came to her eyes and she said 'I just don't feel like I matter.'

How many of us have this feeling or have experienced this feeling? I really, really think that we have got to find this inside ourselves, this feeling that we matter. And the way to that is through self love.

in loving you, i must truly love myself.
for it is in that self love
that i can offer the depths of my
soul to you.

The overlapping of self love and loving others seeps into so many of my thoughts and my meanderings.

"If someone came up to me and asked for my advice on having a healthy, loving relationship, 'acceptance' would probably be the number one thing I'd talk about. That seems to be the thing that is really teaching me love.

Acceptance.

And what's so cool about it is that you can't do it without a TON of self exploration.

You have to figure out why something bugs you. What's YOUR deal with it? Why the reaction? And then you have to figure out if it's something that you can resolve on your own, if you need to go to your partner for help, or if you really need to tweak something between the two of you.

Self responsibility.
Seeing yourself clearly.
Owning your own stuff.
Valuing yourself enough to put it out there if you feel that's the thing to do.
Valuing your partner enough to accept it if that's the correct thing to do.
Respecting your partner enough to allow them to be who they are.

Woe.
There's a ton of things mixed up in this acceptance stuff.
And it's all good and it all leads to healthy individuals and healthy couples.

Yeah, that's where I'd go. Then I'd smile and say, "It'll be harder than you can imagine. Because it's not about your partner. It's about you and what's going on inside of you. If you can figure that out, then you can find acceptance. Acceptance of both you and them."

Maybe that's what I'm figuring out.

Loving someone is so intricately combined with loving yourself that you can't have one without the other."

if i can love you in my heart,
can i carry it down to my bones?
will my cells fill with it,
carrying it past any physical realm?
will i become love when i learn
to really love you?

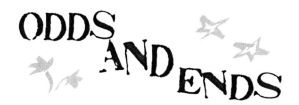

ODDS AND ENDS

There were so many odds and ends, tidbits, a final story (or two) and a stream of consciousness piece that I just wasn't sure how to weave through the book that I decided to make a whole section just for these! What the heck. No particular order here. Just thoughts I wanted to share.

"I'm so excited about this one. See if this makes any sense...

Some ghosts are getting stirred up in me right now. I know why. It makes sense. Or so I thought.

This morning when I walked, some came up. I wanted them to just go away. But maybe I should be doin' something with them if they keep coming back?

I got on my treadmill. Didn't put the music on right away. Thought about this. You know, I think it's not the ghosts but the Terri's that were involved at these moments that I should be focusing on.

These were moments when I felt I needed to keep it all together so I did what I had to do without really taking the time to do anything nurturing for myself.

I think too, I just didn't know what to do for myself. I mean sometimes, you just have to get through and that's okay.

But how about now? When the ghosts keep coming back?

Maybe they're not coming back to haunt you. Maybe they're coming back to nudge you. Tell you it's time to take care of that part of you!

Ohmygosh.

That would change everything.

Instead of telling them to go away, I could ask them where I should look. I could ask them to point the way to healing.

Woe.

I loved this idea, figured walking on the treadmill probably wasn't time to go back and do the nurturing, but I would soon.

I turned the music on and just started doing my thing.

I had the music on random and was just moving along listening when things started happening inside of me.

A song came on about the darkness inside of her.

Oh my gosh. I went right to the darkness inside of me.

I pictured me and my insides that felt dark. I went to the stars I had pictured the other day inside of me. I saw the stars all over me. I just filled up the darkness with stars.

She started singing about 'your mother, your sister, your wife' and I thought of my family I'd be seeing soon and I thought of their ghosts that they had, their hauntings that they dealt with, and I thought they needed some stars.

I'm not sure they remember theirs.

I have plenty.
I can share.

So I pictured different people and I was going around putting stars all around them. I put some gently in their hair, near where they were sitting, just all around them.

I started crying as I was doing this. I'm now running on the treadmill, crying and putting stars everywhere in my mind.

Then some song came on about scars. It's some weird song the guys got me hooked on. The singer names all these scars he's got and where they came from.

Oh my gosh.

He'd list them, I'd picture mine that went with what he was singing and I'd put a star on each one. Some I rubbed the stars gently on, leaving star dust over them. He sang this line about the blood and the rain and never seeing the hurt coming and I was ready to just sob...I nodded to that one.

'I remember blood and rain and I never saw it coming again...'

And yes, the tears were really coming now...

And then! Stevie (my hero, my symbol for following your heart) comes on singing 'Love Struck Baby,' a real fun, kooky falling in love song.

Now I go back to the Ters in the trauma places that I didn't think I should go to while on the treadmill. It doesn't matter. I'm out of control. I'm running to them all with a big grin on my face, singing this kooky love song to them and sprinkling stars on them.

They're all not really in the best place, right? That's why I have to go back to them. They're all really, really struggling.

And I'm running around singing 'Love Struck Baby' dropping stars all around them. I'm rubbing stars on their arms real gently so they can be covered in star dust...

They're liking it. It's helping.

By the time I got off the treadmill I was a sweaty, teary, feeling better mess.

Stevie's lyrics ringing in my ears. 'I'm love struck baby...I must confess...'

This life I've got is so darn cool.

Ghosts...maybe they come with messages.
Ters...maybe I need to hold them more.
Stars...maybe I need to share them. "

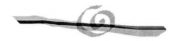

"I had a body chemistry changing moment and MY BODY CHEMISTRY DIDN'T CHANGE! Not only did my body chemistry NOT change, but I handled the moment with grace, ease and best of all, honesty.

Grace.
Ease.
Honesty.

My gosh. What a combination. And no, no, no – NO body chemistry change!

Ha! Ha! Ha! I am toasting this moment.

So I ask myself why? Because I really would like this to be a pattern. I think it's a combination of reasons. Some I won't always get for these moments. But one that I have to pay attention to is this -

I didn't need anything from the person or the moment.

If I don't need anything, then there's no reason for a reaction, is there?

And that, I think, will be one of those wave things. Sometimes I'll have it and sometimes I won't.

And maybe what's important here is that I know that and I cut myself some slack for when I don't do so good.

And I do a little dance with my orange juice when I do!"

"You're only hurting yourself. Remember that trite old comment you heard growing up? You're only hurting yourself. Yeah, yeah, yeah.

Well, I was thinking about that this morning.

I was thinking about the times when we just can't get a concept down for some reason. When we hurt someone over and over again because of our inability to grasp something that we need to grasp. Yes, they get hurt. They also adapt, change, or just look for different things. Maybe they even leave. What happens to us, the ones who aren't getting the concept down? We've lost out. We not only missed the reality of the concept we need to get, we've lost part of that person who is reacting to our missing it. They've shut down to us in that area so we lose part of them, or maybe even all of them.

I saw that real clearly in someone else recently. Oh yeah, always easy to see it somewhere else. So. Now. I had to find it in me. And so I did. Easily. Well, easy to find. Not easy to hold. Ouch. But yeah, I saw real clearly what I'm losing by not getting a concept down. So, time to change that because I'm only hurting myself."

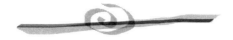

"There are moments here and there when I realize it's still there. I don't carry it everywhere and think of it all the time, it's when the moments that are the hardest for me happen, when I'm doubting myself the most that the feeling surfaces. And that's when I know it's still with me.

How will I ever lose it if it's burned into my cells?

And then it hit me. Maybe you just plain won't, Terri. Maybe you just have to know it's there and reach beyond it.

And then I remembered the branches in the wind this morning. I thought of them reaching high and catching the breeze...maybe you have to do that, Ter. Maybe you have to reach higher and catch the breeze. You are always going to have scars, or branded cells. If it's not this, there will be something else. Because life is full of that stuff. And messages do get burned into cells.

But maybe it's a matter of reaching higher. Which for me, means reaching deeper. Because I think if you reach high enough, deep enough, there's a place where those messages can't hold you back anymore.

Maybe it's not about dropping stuff that you can't drop. Maybe it's about reaching beyond that stuff, and catching the breeze anyway. And letting the breeze carry the weight for you.

Reaching higher.
Reaching deeper.
And riding on the breeze."

144

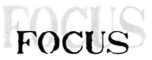

FOCUS

"I'm watching another friend who is discontented right now. And I can see how it's coloring his whole world and causing problems for him.

And so I turned my eyes to my own heart and definitely see discontentment in certain places. When I look at him and his actions, I think of how self centered discontentment makes you. And so I turned my eyes to my own heart again. Yeah, I can be really self centered in my own discontentment.

Amazing how it stunts your vision. And so I kept looking and it brought me back to focusing. Where you focus, what you focus on, what you put your energy towards.

Which brought me to a very short lived friendship that passed through my life. I was feeling bummed that it was so short and gone already. It has been bothering me the last few days. And then I thought of this discontentment and focusing stuff.

Truly, it truly is all in how you look at it.

Everyone I care about passes too quickly through my life. Even if I get years and years and years with them. It's too quick. And yet, I am so lucky to have them come through in the first place.

All these thoughts whirled through the blender of my mind and I whisked them together and got this -

I've got so much. I either concentrate on what I've got and keep working at making it better, expanding my sight as I do so to see everyone involved really clearly, or I look at what I've lost and what I'm missing and focus smaller and smaller and lose the vision.

So, once again, I take my wobbly self down the road remembering I have a gift in my hands."

145

"Had a thought while thinking about someone who's causing a lot of pain. The thought that he just didn't care came through my head. But that's not true, and I knew that. I caught myself and rephrased it to 'He just doesn't care ENOUGH to do something about it.' Hmmm...that actually covers a lot of people I know. Does it cover me? It's got to cover everyone depending on the situation, doesn't it? And so with my biggest challenges in front of me, I asked myself if I cared enough. And I knew that I did.

I realized the work ahead of me if I meant that. And suddenly, I could let these other people who just hadn't seemed to care enough off the hook a bit. I could see the work they'd need to do if they really did care enough. I could understand them not doing it."

~~~~~~~~~~

"How do you find TRUE acceptance? I feel like all I have found is the fake stuff. Or coping skills. In some areas I can find acceptance in part of what's happening, and so I looked at that.

When I have no need, there can be acceptance.
Sometimes.

Although, in some places I clearly have no need and yet can't accept the impact the situation or person has on others. So where does that leave me?

Something did pop into my thoughts this morning – the famous ol' 'live in the moment' thought. It seems to be ONLY when I'm in the moment that I have acceptance. Whew. I really, really wonder if I'll make any progress on this one.

There's a flow. The flow is acceptance. There's more to it. There so much more to that flow, I think. But you have to have acceptance. And it kind of hit me, acceptance is as powerful as gratitude.

I've got the gratitude thing pretty strong. But the acceptance thing, oh not so good. I work on it, but end up doing coping techniques more than any kind of real acceptance. I refocus a lot. And while I think that's invaluable, it's not accepting.

It hit me this morning that this is one of my weakest points. And it's got to be one of the most important points to a full life. Great. Great. But I suppose part of acceptance is accepting that you stink at acceptance and moving on from there.

It's a concept that got renewed respect this morning. Now, what to do about it?"

~~~~~~~~~~

"I pulled him aside before he left. 'You doin' okay? What's bothering you?'

And so we talked. 'I didn't want to come in telling you this was bothering me,' he said.

I looked at him. 'Didn't you know you said it in a hundred different ways tonight?'

No. He didn't know. And I've been thinking about that. Every single one of us does that every single day. What's on our minds and preoccupying our insides is totally coming out in our actions and words. Some people pick it up consciously. Some pick it up and never really understand what they picked up.

There's energy mixing out there. And we're creating a vibe.

So what do we do with that?

There's always going to be stuff bothering us. I think, for me, just sitting down and saying 'this is going on, and this is how I feel' helps me move forward and set it down for a bit and live more in the moment.

I think that's what I need, an acknowledgment of it all. Letting everyone in so they can understand my funkiness, and then knowing that whatever happens is okay. It's a giving permission for the feeling to be there. And then being able to put it down.

Somehow that giving permission is important to me. It changes things. It strangely takes the power away from the feeling.

Maybe what we need is a shelf. A shelf to put things on, to let them be there, to know they're there, to acknowledge them. By placing them there we get some sort of relief and can put them down for a bit and enjoy the other moments.

Maybe we all need to figure out how to make our shelves. Wouldn't it be cool if there was a 'Shelf Building 101' we could all take? And we could learn the best shelf building technique that works for us!

I have to remember that and start a new phrase in my family:

'I just have to build a shelf here, hold this nail, would ya?'

Because for me, I need other people holding the nails. That's part of the whole process."

from her sorrow
she found compassion.
from her grief
she learned understanding.
and from her journey
she became real.

"I decided to do something extra with my walking route as it's just not long enough for me to go to the places in my head I need to go to. So I just changed it to see if I could connect to my inner child a bit more...

Thing is...I connected the second I stepped on the road.
So I think it's more intention and openness than route.

I was knee deep into it with Little Terri when the coolest thing happened... we found a worm.

And I don't know...I'm thinkin' it's cause I was kind of tuned into this kid energy that I stopped. It was goin' the wrong way...goin' AWAY from the nice damp grass into the middle of the dry street where he'd never make it. He'd just shrivel up and die.

I learned this when Josh was a kid. We could never take a walk with him without stopping for the worms. There were some days there were so many worms, we just never walked, we just did worm patrol...he'd toss all the worms back to the cool damp places where they'd survive.

I always let him do the tossin' as I wasn't big into worms and he seemed to have a mission.

But today...I don't know...I was in kid mode.

So there I was, bendin' over this worm actually sayin' out loud 'You're goin' the wrong way, Bud.' I picked him up, which had to feel a little rough to him and tossed him into the grass. I thought of Josh and smiled.

A little ways up the road, there was another. 'Okay, what the heck is with you guys?' I asked it...this was a big one. I stopped and looked at it. 'You're a big fat wise one, aren't ya?' and yes, the worm conversations were out loud. At least my part of them was.

I picked him up and tossed him into the grass. I noticed I wasn't as gentle with him. He's big and fat, he can handle the toss...

And then...yep...you guessed it...there was another.

This was a tiny one. Ohh, just a little guy. I very very gently picked him up and tossed him lightly over to the grass.

Almost home when I saw a worm goin' the right way! He was headin' straight into the place that would make him thrive! He did, however, have a fair distance to go. But I didn't stop to help him. I knew he'd make it...it would take him awhile...but he'd do okay.

I turned into my driveway thinking about the worms...what if, Ms. Ter, you were like those worms...you were headin' directly in a direction that would dry you out and make you whither...what if you got picked up and tossed completely into another spot?

What would you do?

I'd grumble. I'd complain. I'd say 'Ouch!' a lot. And I may even spend a good bit of time tryin' to get back to where I started with which was wrong in the first place.

Hmm...

And the tosses?

When the worm was tiny and small, the toss was more gentle...when the worm was big and fat and wise...it was one heck of a toss...he could handle it.

Hmmmmm...maybe there's a lesson in the worms for me this morning.

I don't think I've ever said 'thank you' to whatever force tossed me into a new direction before...well, that's not true...I have said thank you...but it took me years to figure it out. Years later I knew it had been a good thing.

What if you knew right when you landed.
Splat.
That it was a good thing.

What if you KNEW?"

STREAM OF CONSCIOUSNESS

tilting her head back, she asked.
laying in the sun, she asked.
mowing the lawn, she asked.
grocery shopping, she asked.
zipping their coats, she asked.
washing their dishes, she asked.
at parties, at events, at picnics, at concerts, at family gatherings,
on the phone, over email, in her letters, she asked.
ignite. bam. whoosh. shatter.
her answer exploded in her face.
her answer exploded in her veins.
her answer exploded in her heart.
her answer exploded in her soul.
the earth collapsed and covered her. people ran away.
the real ones stayed. stood by with shovels.
the kids. what about the kids?
who takes care of them in an earthquake?
their needs moved the earth for her.
the top layers anyway.
standing up, still covered, but moving, she did what she had to do.
no time for shovels yet.
make the sandwiches, read the books, talk about their feelings.
walk to the woods and cry.
cover her head at night and cry.
make breakfast and believe.
make lunch murmuring to herself.
"everything i need is inside me."
over and over and over and over and over and over and over and over.
spread your fingers wide. release them.
let them go.
spread your fingers wide. release them again.
scream in the car where no one can hear.
stay quiet when they're listening.
close the door and let it out.
anger fills you.
eat my dust.
anger fuels you.
believe you can do it.
know you can do it.

you can do it.
there is no choice.
you will do it.
make their dinner. wash their dishes.
figure out numbers. pray to god.
ask the universe.
do it.
stay up at night and do what must be done.
get up early and do some more.
feel the sand under your eyelids.
try to laugh and see the light.
gather your courage.
swallow your pride.
go door to door.
sell yourself.
i can't do this.
you have to do this.
they'll take them.
you've got a deal.
phone calls ring.
our very first fax.
stomach knots on bill paying day.
checks coming in just when we need it.
guys, we need this much money.
guys, we got this much money.
it worked.
we did it.
the universe listened.
we danced.
we cried.
they leaned on my door and forgave me.
i cried.
i leaned on my door and still couldn't forgive me.
we grew.
they became men.
early.
cars got fixed.
websites got built.
plumbing, electrical, roofing, painting, digging, mechanical,
we can do it all. we have google. we have muscles. we have will.
i'm scared.
hold on.

we're a team.
air compressors proved it.
we became unstoppable.
he watched.
he helped.
he read schematics for long periods of time and understood them.
he read me for long periods of time and sometimes understood me.
we gathered round him.
we can help.
your kids just need love.
we gave and gave and gave and gave and gave.
we must believe it did good that we will never see.
there was hurt and hurt and hurt some more.
we stepped back.
he stepped closer.
i stepped closer.
we laughed.
we hurt.
i cried.
we committed.
except for the dogs. it's still a partial thing we have to hurdle.
but it's not. and we both know it.
the shovels have been out for years now.
digging is routine.
a way of life.
accepted and okay.
the kids are men.
they know pain, they know psychology,
and they love me anyway.
one's moved further on.
two thinking about their own flights.
stuff whirls up again.
open you fingers and release.
open your fingers and let them go.
they aren't now.
you need to know.
he's not them.
they're not you.
love is there.
you found your way.
and you're moving forward.

the new door wouldn't open
with the old key –
she found scrubbing the key
wasn't enough.
she needed a brand new one.

"I'm taking my spirit back. Not sure how. But I know darn sure I'm not living without it."

~~~

"Control is just another way of covering your eyes and when you get really way into the control freak stuff, you've blinded yourself. So, in my mind, a life worth living has to be filled with seeing."

~~~

"Your soul cannot be alive without gratitude. I believe that with my whole heart."

~~~

"Offering to the world when you're hurting...being able to offer compassion and kindness with your unique gifts mixed in while you are struggling and hurting...well, shoot, that's the stuff that keeps your heart open. And I'm thinking that's the stuff that changes the world."

~~~

"Over and over again I am reminded of the power we have in the tiniest of acts. Our responses all through the day mean more than we choose to know. I am committed to watch my responses and be aware of the potential of each one."

~~~

"And then he said it...'Maybe you just don't ever have it until you really believe you do.'
Ohhh...I paused and said real low...'Maybe that's with everything.'
'Yeah, maybe it is,' he said."

~~~

"Don't look for what people can't give you."

"Best thing that happened to me yesterday – I was overcome by a deep sense of compassion for MYSELF."

~~~

"I want to feel it. I don't want to close down. I don't want to fill with fear. I just want to feel."

~~~

"This morning as I walked through all the puddles of tears, there was a crispness in the air. It's both. It's puddles and puddles of tears and the hope of a new day in the air."

~~~

"The stuff I was/am angry about and frustrated with is still there. But my heart moved. I still have anger. If I dwell on it, I can feel the anger. The choice is not to dwell on it. That's my choice right now. It's where I dwell, I guess. And who knows...in a few hours anger or sadness may overtake me. I wouldn't be surprised if it did. And if it does, then maybe I can use it and watch. Because it's in the watching that I'm learning. And it's in the learning that I'm growing. And it's in the growing that I'm becoming."

~~~

"I guess it would be a 'balance' thing. If I can protect my heart, but leave it open to me...well, then, maybe that would be the way of choice at times."

~~~

"An after thought that has me intrigued...what's so important about the little things is the ACT of doing them. Good or bad."

~~~

"I felt something go through me. A feeling. A thought. Yeah, it's all a game. The whole thing is a game. There's sad parts and hard parts and traumatic parts and joyful parts and goofy parts and satisfying parts...and it's all a game. I could hear the whisper, 'Come play with me.' I looked up at the sky, bowed down to it and said, 'Okay, I'll play.'"

" I can't do it.
Beep.
Wrong.
I WON'T do it.
Think I'd better claim that one. This is a choice I'm making. And right away that felt powerful. Because WHY am I making it? Hmmmmm..."

~~~

"We talked about the people who REALLY knew their stuff and didn't put it in your face. I added that it seemed to me that the really talented people are the ones who can offer admiration easily. I have found that the people who come to me and compliment me the most are people who are so out of my league in talent, yet they share admiration for me anyway."

~~~

I want to learn the balance. Learn the balance of holding things, feeling feelings, hurting and knowing that it's not all that bad. I want to learn the balance of feeling the sad and letting it be there without having it take my whole life away with it."

~~~

"Behind good communication is more than just saying the words the other person can hear in a way they can hear. It's the ability to know HOW they hear. It's the wanting to know how they hear and how they process. It's the strength to reach out when you're exhausted in a way that's not natural for you, but is the way that they'll hear. That, to me, is essential in a relationship."

~~~

"There's always something I'm trying to hurdle, walk through, or hide from! It occurs to me that somewhere down deep I was thinking if I got far enough, I wouldn't have to be doing this hurdling, walking, or hiding any more. What was I thinking??? It's a lifetime of that stuff. So get used to it. Make it an accepted part of your life, Ter. Not something that you fight all the time."

"It's not about pushing to be more, is it? We don't have to be more. We have 'it' already. Stop the pushing and just be. Breathe it in and know it. Breathe it out and live it."

~~~

"I came into my studio and threw open the windows. I'm letting the sky in today! Because it's just so big I think it needs to leak out everywhere this morning. I'm going to fill my heart with it and carry it with me all day. It's going to leak out my eyes. People are going to say 'Ohhhh your eyes are so blue, why I do believe they're SKY BLUE today!' I'll smile and nod and say 'Why yes, I do believe they are.' And me and the sky, well, we'll know what's going on."

-and she turned to find the sky inside her.

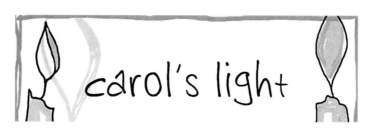

carol's light

It had taken a long time, months, I guess, for me to get back to a spot where I really felt okay about business again. I'd make progress and then lose it, and then do okay and be kind of steady, but not really. Finally, finally, I felt not only steady, I felt really good about things. Not because any money was rolling in. Oh no, no real practical reason. There was just a coming back to that knowing that I'm going in the right direction, just feeling solid inside, in my bones. I had finally reached this spot. Hadn't been there very long at all when something happened that touched me in a thousand different ways.

I got a note from a shop owner I work with. Dani's become more than someone I work with, she's become a friend. She had told me about one of her customers named Carol. Carol had liked the bone sighs a lot, joked about needing a twelve step program for her addiction to them, and apparently was one of our most loyal customers.

Dani wrote me one morning that Carol had suddenly and unexpectedly died. She told me that just recently Carol had actually said that when she died she wanted to be buried with a bone sigh in her hand – along with her pink fishing pole! As I read the note, I cried.

After writing Dani back, I turned to my desk. There were a million things going on that day. But I didn't care. I just stopped everything. I wanted to write a bone sigh for Carol. I didn't know her. Just had a passing exchange of emails. But I was so filled with wanting to do something to honor her. I could just feel it and wanted to let that flow.

I turned to write. But it's about death. I'm not real good with death. I try to be. I try to be all okay with it and accepting...but I'm not really there yet. I have no real beliefs of what happens after you die. Are you around and watching us or are you just gone or what? I just don't know. I realized my lack of beliefs when my dad died. I never had a feeling like he was there around me. It was glaringly obvious that I had no particular belief to hold on to. I didn't know what I thought about it all and have been shaky ever since. So the writing of this bone sigh wasn't working quite right. I scribbled a few things, didn't like them, kept trying. Finally I stopped.

I sat still. I thought of Carol. I wondered where she was. This act was completely for her. I had no other motivation but to honor her. Where was she now? Was there any chance she could be around? I looked out the window. 'You nearby?' I asked. 'Wanna help?'

I honestly have no idea if she was around or not. I just left it entirely open. And I turned back to the paper. And this time I wrote from a whole different angle. I wrote as if it was Carol talking to her best friend who loved her and was aching with missing her. I wrote what she would say to her. I hadn't had this angle before, it was completely different than the other directions I was taking. But it felt really good. It felt right. I just wrote it down and was done. Okay, I thought. That's what it will be. I turned to do the art and get it all together. I wanted to put it together fast and get it back from the printer quickly so that I could ship it out to the shop owner. She could give them away to people she thought could use them.

As I was putting the art with the words, I felt a lot of self doubt. I hadn't felt any when I was writing, but now that I was trying to put it together to finalize, I started doubting. I wanted it to be right. I wanted to honor Carol in a way that really worked.

I sent a digital image to Dani, told her what I was up to and told her I was having some self doubts. She replied with hearty encouragement and told me to tell the doubts to 'kiss off.' I knew the doubts didn't matter, that I had to do this because everything inside of me was telling me so. I nodded in agreement to her note. I told her I would be shipping her some in a few days.

The next morning, she wrote again. She had a story for me. She was in her shop doing her shopkeeper duties, when a woman came in and stopped at the bone sigh display. She held a print in her hand and was crying. Dani's not just a shop owner, she's a woman with a mission. She wants to touch people and love them and live a life of this stuff. She walked up to the woman and started talking to her. Dani's also a great writer, and in her note to me, she pulled me into the story of her conversation with this woman and how she discovered that Carol was this woman's best friend! How they had recently spent the afternoon together and had such fun. How when they had said goodbye that day they agreed to do that kind of thing more often, and now she was gone. She cried as she told all this to Dani.

Dani described the scene to me, she told me of wrapping her arms around her, telling her one arm was from Dani and one arm was from me. She told her that I had just designed a bone sigh in Carol's honor and was sending them up. Julie sobbed as she heard this.

As I read this note, I was crying pretty good myself. I couldn't believe it. I had written that bone sigh for Julie. I knew that as I read the note. Whether Carol was guiding me, or my inner voice was guiding me, or just some deep connections were doing the guiding...I didn't care. All I knew was that by listening, I was led. I saw the connections between Dani, and Carol, and Julie and me. I saw the power of reaching out in love. From Dani's touching this woman's arm and talking to her, to Julie's going to the shop reaching for something, to my listening to my heart.

I cried for Julie's loss in her best friend, for the loss of a woman who touched so many lives, for the beauty of Dani's heart, and for being so powerfully reminded to listen to my own. I had come back to that knowing just a day or two before this all happened. This felt like an affirmation that was so big I didn't even know what to do with it. I haven't put it down yet.

And then there's Carol, a woman who died suddenly and unexpectedly. It happens every day. All the time. Will I have lived the life that I wanted when I'm at the end of my own journey? I so want that answer to be yes. The only way that I know that I will be able to say that is if I keep listening to that voice inside of me and following my heart.

carol's light

tears flowing, face scrunched in pain,
i ask out loud 'what would she say now?'
the answer whispers inside me,
'i haven't left you. i'm in your heart.
feel me loving you. that hasn't stopped.
listen for me when you need me -
and remember i am part of you.'
placing my hand on my heart,
i closed my eyes and felt her.

161

she laced up her dancing shoes every day.
opening her heart
as she did so.
stepping into the all,
she kicked up her feet,
touched the stars,
and danced with life.

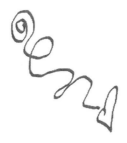

Terri is an author and artist and owner of her home based business, bone sigh arts. She's just about finished raising her three sons and feels she has been growing up right along side of them. For her last birthday, she was gifted with a brand new bike complete with star streamers coming out of the handlebars! She's noticed that when she rides early in the morning, and those streamers of stars fly through the air at a certain angle, the sky begins to talk to her. 'Sometimes it's shouting so joyfully to me, reminding me that my heart is as limitless as the sky itself, and sometimes it's whispering to me to just release and trust. And always, always it's reminding me that I am loved.' You can find her in the mornings, talking to the sky.

Want to learn more?

Come on over to bone sigh arts at www.BoneSighArts.com.
Or visit Terri's blog at www.BoneSighArts.blogspot.com.
Find more books at www.BoneSighBooks.com

Love that cover art?

Visit Graphic Designer, Noah Urban, at wwwBFGproductions.com

CPSIA information can be obtained
at www.ICGtesting.com
Printed in the USA
FFOW04n1032061014
7814FF